Digital and
Radiographic
Imaging

For Elsevier:

Commissioning Editor: Claire Wilson
Development Editor: Catherine Jackson
Project Manager: Christine Johnston
Designer: Erik Bigland

Digital and Radiographic Imaging

A PRACTICAL APPROACH

Fourth Edition

Chris Gunn MA TDCR

CGTraining, Retford, Nottinghamshire, UK

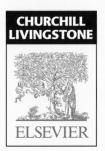

CHURCHILL LIVINGSTONE

ELSEVIER

EDINBURGH LONDON NEW YORK OXFORD PHILADELPHIA ST LOUIS SYDNEY TORONTO 2009

CHURCHILL
LIVINGSTONE
ELSEVIER

ELSEVIER your source for books,
journals and multimedia
in the health sciences
www.elsevierhealth.com

First edition 1988
Second edition 1994
Third edition 2002
Fourth edition 2009

ISBN: 978-0-443-06863-8

British Library Cataloguing in Publication Data
A catalogue record for this book is available from the British
Library

Library of Congress Cataloging in Publication Data
A catalog record for this book is available from the Library of
Congress

Notice
Knowledge and best practice in this field are constantly changing.
As new research and experience broaden our knowledge,
changes in practice, treatment and drug therapy may become
necessary or appropriate. Readers are advised to check the most
current information provided (i) on procedures featured or (ii) by
the manufacturer of each product to be administered, to verify the
recommended dose or formula, the method and duration of
administration, and contraindications. It is the responsibility of the
practitioner, relying on their own experience and knowledge of the
patient, to make diagnoses, to determine dosages and the best
treatment for each individual patient, and to take all appropriate
safety precautions. To the fullest extent of the law, neither the
Publisher nor the Author assumes any liability for any injury
and/or damage to persons or property arising out or related to
any use of the material contained in this book. *The Publisher*

Working together to grow
libraries in developing countries

www.elsevier.com | www.bookaid.org | www.sabre.org

ELSEVIER   BOOK AID
International   Sabre Foundation

The
publisher's
policy is to use
**paper manufactured
from sustainable forests**

Printed in China

Contents

Seven years ago, when editing the third edition of this book, I wrote that '. . . computers have become commonplace in imaging departments, and advances with regard to Picture Archiving and Communication Systems (PACS), the advent of the Digital Imaging and Communication in Medicine project (DICOM) and the introduction of image analysis has meant that their future is assured. In spite of that, many departments still use conventional films and cassettes and therefore I have retained the more traditional aspects of radiographic imaging.' I was expecting therefore that by the time this edition was being written, films, cassettes and processing would be obsolete and would no longer be included in this book. In the UK and much of Europe, this is virtually the case, with the exception of mammography and dental radiography in dental practices; but after having conversations with manufacturers' representatives, I have discovered that there are still hospitals in China, Africa and India that have not yet 'gone digital'. As this book has worldwide sales, I decided, therefore, to change the format of the whole book to a more user-friendly note format, expand the digital side and include the basic imaging principles for ultrasound, CT scanning, MRI and nuclear medicine and retain the 'conventional processing' information in the Appendices.

The pace of change is such that virtually no textbook is able to keep up with the advances in technology. Fortunately, much of the information is now available on the internet and, for that reason, I have included details of manufacturers' websites, as opposed to more traditional references. These sites are kept up-to-date by the manufacturers and provide a valuable source of additional information on new products. I have included any direct sources or articles at the end of the appropriate chapter.

Derrick Roberts and Nigel Smith were the original authors of *Radiographic Imaging*, and I was privileged to listen to both of them lecture on the practical aspects of photography. Their extensive knowledge on the subject provided a sound basis for this book and their hard work must be acknowledged as they provided the foundation for this present edition.

Finally, I would like to thank the manufacturers who sent me literature and those who keep their very comprehensive websites up-to-date. It is very clear that all of us could no longer manage without computers, and the information they provide and their ability to transfer information throughout the health community can only be of benefit to patients.

Chris Gunn
Retford 2009

It is often argued that radiography is more art than science. Whilst the argument has never been settled, it is indisputable that a great deal of radiography requires a practical approach.

This book has been written to satisfy the need for more practical knowledge in the imaging sciences. To this end every chapter, wherever possible, connects the theory with the practice.

The book is aimed at students in the field of diagnostic imaging, from graduate and postgraduate radiographic students to trainee radiologists. The book can be of use as a reference within the imaging department and as a manual of photographic quality assurance and fault finding which is easy to understand and read.

Particular attention has been paid to the subject areas where our experience has indicated most of the common misconceptions occur. The science of imaging is too complex a subject to be covered by one book. If further information is required in specialised areas, the reader is referred to other experts in the field.

It should be added that the interpretations expressed in this book are our own and may conflict with the long-standing opinions of others.

D. P. Roberts
N. L. Smith

HOW COMPUTERS WORK

<table>
<tr><td></td><td>

Keyboard
Each key represents a number of electrical signals (a stream of electrons and spaces)

To input data
A key is depressed

For each key depressed
A number of electrical impulses (signals and non-signals) are sent to the computer

Silicon chip
The circuits on the silicon chips are activated

Signal
A corresponding signal is sent to the screen (composed of signals and non-signals)

Image formation
When an electron interacts with the screen the screen fluoresces
When there are no electrons it does not fluoresce

Example image of a letter T
111111
00**11**00
00**11**00   Where 0 = no electron
00**11**00   and 1 = electron

</td></tr>
<tr><td>

Decimal System

</td><td>

- To base 10
- Each column represents an increase by a factor of 10, e.g. ten (10), hundred (100), thousand (1000), etc.
- This system is too complex for computers to handle in this format

</td></tr>
<tr><td>

Binary

</td><td>

- To base 2
- Each column represents an increase by a factor of 2, e.g. two (2), four (4), eight (8), sixteen (16), thirty two (32), sixty four (64), etc.

A	64	32	16	8	4	2	1	= Decimal numbers
B	1	1	1	0	1	1	0	= Binary number
C	0	1	0	1	0	0	1	= Binary number

</td></tr>
<tr><td>

To Change Binary to Decimal
(This can be done automatically by using a computer's Scientific Calculator)

</td><td>

Example 1
- Take row B above and read off the corresponding numbers in row A
- = 64, 32, 16, 4, 2
- Add the numbers together = 118
- Therefore 1110110 = 118

Example 2
- Take row C above and read off the corresponding numbers in row A
- 32, 8, 1
- Add the numbers together = 41
- Therefore 0101001 = 41

</td></tr>
<tr><td>

To Change Decimal to Binary
(This can be done automatically by using a computer's Scientific Calculator)

</td><td>

128   64   32   16   8   4   2   1

Example
To change 118 to Binary
- 118 is smaller than 128 therefore = **0**
- 118 is larger than 64 therefore = **1** (118 − 64 = 54)
- 54 is larger than 32 therefore = **1** (54 − 32 = 22)
- 22 is larger than 16 therefore = **1** (22 − 16 = 6)
- 6 is smaller than 8 therefore = **0**
- 6 is larger than 4 therefore = **1** (6 − 4 = 2)
- 2 is the same as 2 therefore = **1** (2 − 2 = 0)
- 0 is smaller than 1 therefore = **0**
The binary number is therefore **01110110**

(continued on next page)

</td></tr>
</table>

HOW COMPUTERS WORK *continued*	
Bit (BInary digiT)	• The smallest piece of information that a computer can handle • Represented by a simple electrical signal • Which is either ON or OFF • 0 represents OFF • 1 represents ON
Byte	• Equals 8 bits • Can represent numbers 0 to 255 inclusive • Which is 256 different combinations of ON and OFF • The main use for the numbers 0 to 255 is in the ASCII code (The American Standard Code for Information Exchange) to designate numbers, characters and symbols used on the computer keyboard *Example* [Decimal] [Binary] [Character] 115 01110011 s 34 00100010 " 68 01000100 D
Hexadecimal System	• To the base 16 • Using numbers 0 to 9 and letters A to F • Therefore representing large (decimal or binary numbers) with fewer characters • Conversion can be done automatically by using a computer's Scientific Calculator up to a maximum of 16 digits using Qword option **Table 1.1** **Comparison of decimal, hexadecimal and binary number systems 0–20**

Decimal	Hexadecimal	Binary
0	0	0
1	1	1
2	2	10
3	3	11
4	4	100
5	5	101
6	6	110
7	7	111
8	8	1000
9	9	1001
10	A	1010
11	B	1011
12	C	1100
13	D	1101
14	E	1110
15	F	1111
16	10	10000
17	11	10001
18	12	10010
19	13	10011
20	14	10100

SILICON CHIPS

Components	• A rectangle of silicon (the wafer), forming the base and part of the electrical connection • 4 or 5 square centimetres (cm) in size • A layer of active components – containing up to one thousand million transistors • A layer of passive components – wires • Round the edge are pads of metal – forming connections • The layers (or features) are 65–90 nanometres (nm) thick

(continued on next page)

SILICON CHIPS *continued*

The Silicon Chip (Microchip)	• Microchips are printed, using a form of photography, through a photo-resist (light sensitive material) and directly onto the chip material
	• The final resolution of this process is produced by reducing a large negative to a microscopically small size
	• Originally used ultraviolet light as the printing light: giving a final resolution of 1/1000 of a millimetre (mm)
	• If beams of electrons are used the resolution is doubled
	• Heavy ion imaging produces finer detail and permits 'ballistic transfer' of electrons, on a very small chip
	  ○ Ballistic transfer means that the distances within the chip are so small that the electrons travel like bullets to their destination, without even atoms intervening into their path
	• The resultant changes in the photo-resist are removed by a solvent
	  ○ In a Positive photo-resist the parts exposed are removed
	  ○ In a Negative photo-resist the unexposed parts are removed

COMPUTER LANGUAGES

Machine Code	**Historically** • Computer inputs and outputs were on paper tape • Involved calculations • Instructions were turned into binary arithmetic (machine code)
High Level Languages	• A language in which each instruction or statement (in almost plain English) corresponds to several machine code instructions • The most common of the high level languages has become BASIC, initiated by *Microsoft* • BASIC has many dialects, therefore a program written in one dialect of BASIC will not run on another dialect of BASIC
BASIC Reserve Words (Examples in BOLD)	To enable any computer to **RUN** it must have some form of language for it to be able to **LOAD** a program. You may wish to **SAVE** the program onto disk or tape. It may also be necessary in the program for the computer to **READ** a set of **DATA** and, from time to time, **GOTO** various sections of the program to be able to **LIST** certain variables which have been turned into **STRING**s. You may also have to **WAIT WHILE** the computer **WEND**s its way through very long **CHAIN**s of numbers before it can **RESTORE** itself and **RETURN** to the program and allow you to **INPUT** more information before it will **PRINT** out the name you wanted to **DELETE**. Eventually the program will **STOP, END** and finally **CLOSE**. • Give a computer specific instructions as to what to do • The Universal language among home computers, mainly due to the simplicity of programming • Unsuitable for large scale programming as, it is very slow as all the instructions have to be translated into machine code by the computer • Programs, written in BASIC are not *portable*, i.e. they will *not* run on a different machine
Syntax (Programme construction or rules)	• When programming, exact reserve words and punctuation must be used or the program will not run, e.g. GOTO can only be entered as GOTO, not GO TO • A comma (,) a colon (:) or double quotes (") are also used
CP/M (A standard 'business' computer language)	• Any computer capable of running CP/M is capable of running any program written in that language
DICOM (Digital Imaging and Communications in Medicine)	This is a communications protocol to enable standardisation in medical data files produced and updated by the National Electrical Manufacturers Association (NEMA). **Aim** • To integrate information and management systems so that clinical information can be communicated among all specialities and providers • Allow images and data to be exchanged between computers and hospitals

(continued on next page)

COMPUTER LANGUAGES *continued*

DICOM *(contd)*	• Any doctor will eventually have access to a wide range of tests and images, on computer
	• The primary concern is patient confidentiality
	It is essential that:
	• Passwords and security systems are regularly reviewed
	• A system of monitoring the access to each piece of information and producing an audit trail of when the information is accessed, for how long and by using which password is used
	• All new systems are checked to ensure that they are using DICOM and can be updated
	  ○ DICOM Standards are updated four or five times each year
	  ○ Re-published at least every 2 years

The Problems	**Image files**
	• Contain coded data for each pixel that forms the image
	• Contain a header file, which
	  ○ Contains instructions on how to decode the image
	  ○ This file must be recognised by the system originating the image and the one receiving it
	  ○ If the file is not recognised it cannot be read

Standard File Formats	• The computer language the file is written in should be a standard language • Tagged Information File Format (TIFF) is one of the most common formats • Therefore a TIFF file can be reliably read by most software
Computer Operating Systems	• Include systems such as Windows or DOS • Problems occur if an optical disk is written by equipment from one manufacturer and cannot be read on the system of another manufacturer • DICOM introduces standard operating system protocols to reduce this problem
Networks	• Computers on the same network can transfer files • Problems can happen when trying to transfer files to another network • DICOM introduces standard network protocols to prevent this problem • File transfer protocol (FTP) tends to be the protocol of choice

The System	• Identifies a set of standards
	• Used by all DICOM compliant manufacturers
	• Systems from different manufacturers can communicate with each other
	• The system is made up of fields
	• Each system has specific information attached as an Application Entity Title (AET), e.g.:
	  ○ Specific hospital
	  ○ Imaging system (MRI, ultrasound, CT, etc.)
	• Information associated with each image file and how it is formatted is specified
	• Information objects specify how images from different modalities communicate with each other, e.g.:
	  ○ Outlines what information is contained about the patient (given name, surname, etc.)
	  ○ Object class definition explains the reason for the file, e.g. patient information
	• Network operations deal with networking protocols

The Manufacturer	• Has to produce a compliance statement for each piece of equipment; this should be available to anyone purchasing that equipment and includes:
	  ○ How the system interacts with communications from a third party
	  ○ Determines the DICOM capabilities of the equipment

Service Classes	• Service classes contain protocols for linking with other systems, e.g. Electronic Health Record Systems or Radiology Information Systems (RIS) with regard to:
	  ○ Producing images
	  ○ Processing images
	  ○ Image display
	  ○ Image retrieval
	  ○ Sending images
	  ○ Image printing

(continued on next page)

COMPUTER LANGUAGES *continued*

Service Classes (*contd*)	○ Image storage
	○ Image queries
	• Service class users (SCU)
	  ○ Send out information specific to that equipment
	• Service class providers (SCP)
	  ○ Store images specific to that equipment

Advantages of DICOM	• Allows the integration of network hardware, servers, scanners, printers, workstations from different manufacturers • Better access to images • Time saving – information has only to be entered once • Allows different manufactures equipment to 'talk' to each other • Can link with other medical systems (pathology, dermatology, etc.) non-imaging modalities and information systems
Disadvantages of DICOM	• Not all manufacturers fully support DICOM

SOURCES

Patefield S 1996a DICOM explained. Synergy, March
Patefield S 1996b What is DICOM and why is it so important? Synergy, May

TYPES OF HARDWARE

Computer	A device for processing information quickly and easily, and comes in many shapes and sizes

Computer Types	**Mainframe**
	A large computer, usually the centre of a system. Intelligent peripherals can then be attached to this.
	
	Personal computer (PC)
	A general purpose machine that enables the user to perform a number of tasks including using word processing, spreadsheets, databases, e-mail, internet access
	• **Desktop computers** used in a permanent position usually have a:
	  ○ Tower that holds the computer
	  ○ A monitor
	  ○ A separate keyboard
	  ○ A mouse
	• **Laptop small computer** usually contains everything in one box:
	  ○ Computer, monitor and touch screen
	• **Personal Digital Assistant** (e.g. a 'Blackberry') A small, handheld, wireless computer which performs all the tasks of a personal computer

Main Parts	**Central Processing Unit (CPU)**
	The microprocessor that controls the working of the computer in the three main areas of:
	• The memory
	  ○ Area used to hold data
	• The arithmetic logic
	  ○ Performs mathematical calculations, including logic functions
	• Control unit
	  ○ Fetches information
	  ○ Stores the information
	  ○ Interprets the information
	
	Hard disk
	Permanent store for:
	• Programs
	• Files
	• Documents, etc.
	
	Operating system
	Integral software
	• Allows the operator to communicate with the computer
	
	Power supply
	Electricity is supplied via a step-down transformer

Types of Memory	**Random Access Memory (RAM)** Temporarily stores the information the computer is working with • Where a program is loaded when it is being used • The higher the RAM the faster the computer will work **Read Only Memory (ROM)** A permanent memory store • It cannot be changed and remains when the computer is switched off • Used for basic information that does not change **Basic input/output system** Used when the computer is switched on • Establishes the basic connections **Virtual memory** A temporary data store on the hard drive • Interacts with RAM when required

(continued on next page)

TYPES OF HARDWARE *continued*

Circuit Boards	**Motherboard** Main circuit board of a computer • Holds the CPU and the Memory **Sound card** Used to record and play audio • Converts analogue sound to digital information • And digital information to analogue **Graphics card** Used to display images on the monitor **Network card** Used to enable one computer to directly connect with another via a network connection
Interfaces	**Integrated Drive Electronics (IDE)** The main interface between: • The hard drive and the disk drive **Peripheral Component Interconnect (PCI)** Slots into the motherboard • A common method of connecting additional components, e.g. additional memory cards **Small Computer System Interface (SCSI)** Means of adding additional devices, e.g. scanners **Accelerated Graphics Port (AGP)** A high speed connection • Enables the graphics card to interface with the computer
Connections	**Input/outputs** The interaction between the computer and the components • Monitor – displays information (see Monitor Technology p. 21) • Keyboard – main method for entering information • Removable storage – DVDs, etc. (see Image Storage p. 45) **Ports** 'Sockets' • Parallel – usually used to connect a printer • Serial – usually used to connect an external modem • Universal Serial Bus (USB) – most common external connection used to connect: ○ A mouse, printers, etc. **Networks** External communications enabling multiway communication • **Local Area Network (LAN)** a method of connecting computers in the same area (see Computer Networking p. 53) • **Intranet** a network of computers within a specific area, e.g. a hospital or group of hospitals • **PACS** **P**icture **A**rchiving and **C**ommunications **S**ystem, for allowing transfer of images and data across the intranet, e.g. radiographs and reports • **Healthlink** a centralised, data communications network, which enables authorised users to exchange documents and information **Modem** (**MO**dulator-**DEM**odulator). A device, or interface, also known as an acoustic coupler • Means of connecting a computer to the internet
Accessories	**Mouse** Equipment to navigate round a computer monitor and to interact with it • It makes the computer more 'user friendly' • It is used by rolling the device across a desk top which, moves a cursor to icon displays on the screen

(continued on next page)

TYPES OF HARDWARE *continued*

Accessories (*contd*)	**Touch screen**
	A type of mouse found on laptop computers
	• Controlled by finger tip pressure on the screen
	
	Printers
	• Inkjet printer
	  ◦ Ink is sprayed on to paper through very fine jets
	  ◦ Characters or images are built in very fine dots virtually silently
	  ◦ Typically resolutions of 300×300 d.p.i. (dots per inch) can be expected
	  ◦ Some ink cartridges contain the printhead
	• Laser printer
	  ◦ Does not use ink cartridges but 'toner'
	  ◦ The characters or images are built up by being scanned by a laser and then toner is fused onto the paper
	  ◦ Resolution (up to 600×600 d.p.i.)
	
	Scanner
	A device which enables documents, pictures, etc. to be scanned
	• The resultant scan is held as a digital image

Communicating with a Computer	**Light pen**
	A device, shaped like a pen, which interfaces with a computer screen to enable writing, drawing or to click menu buttons. Enables signatures to be recorded on computer documents
	
	Speech recognition
	Software, allowing computers to be operated by human voice commands
	
	Speech synthesis
	Software allowing the computer to 'talk' to the user
	
	Barcode reader
	A barcode is a series of black and white parallel lines of varying thickness, each line representing a number. These can be scanned by either:
	• Using a light beam
	  ◦ The reflected beam is detected by a charge-coupled device
	  ◦ The analogue signal is converted to a digital signal
	• Or a laser beam
	  ◦ Works as the light beam
	  ◦ Can be used at a larger distance
	  ◦ Is more expensive
	The information is then decoded by the computer and therefore in the hospital situation, patient identification information can be produced as a bar code and when scanned automatically added to the appropriate field on the screen

TYPES OF SOFTWARE

Software	**Software** The programs run by the computer **Firmware** Software stored on a chip
Operating System	**Disk Operating System (DOS)** The software which controls the disk drive **Access time** The time taken for the computer to get information from a storage device, e.g. disk or tape **Analogue** Represents a quantity changing in steps which are continuous, i.e. a sine wave, as opposed to *digital* which is in discrete steps **Analogue to digital convertor** A device which converts analogue signals into digital signals which can be understood by the computer **Arithmetic logic unit** Area responsible for logic and mathematical calculations **Baud** The unit for measuring the rate at which data is transmitted or received **Bits per second (bps)** The rate information is transferred between computers **Booting** The action of starting up the computer by loading it with its starting instructions **Buffer** An area which stores information at one rate and releases it at a slower rate to another device, e.g. a buffer can be sited between a computer (fast) and a printer (which is significantly slower). Data can then be passed at a fast rate and stored in the buffer until the printer can print the data, therefore the computer is freed for further work much more rapidly **Characters per second (CPS)** A measure of the speed of data output **Chip** A piece of silicon or gallium arsenide which contains the microcircuitry which operates the computer **Dot matrix** A square or rectangle of dots which, given instructions by the computer, forms a character on the screen **Download** To transfer information from one computer to another **FAQ** **F**requently **A**sked **Q**uestion **Gate** The basis of all computer operations and performs a single logical operation when subjected to a number of inputs **Graphical User Interface (GUI)** Enables the operator to use the computer intuitively via graphics (pictures) showing programs to run, directories they are kept in etc., e.g. 'Windows' from Microsoft **Graphics** • Computerised 'drawing', known as CAD (Computer Aided Drawing or Design) • The ability of the computer to produce preprogrammed graphic characters • The mode the computer has to be placed in prior to drawing graphics

(continued on next page)

TYPES OF SOFTWARE *continued*	
Operating System (*contd*)	**Graphics tablet** Equipment that can digitise drawing or graphs ready for input into the computer **Handshake** An electronic signal which indicates the end of the passage of data from the computer
Word Processing	A combination of computer, software and printer enabling the user to produce high quality text which can be manipulated electronically before being committed to paper
Spreadsheet	A program which allows forecasting and financial planning if any variable is altered. The effects throughout the program can be demonstrated and the figures changed throughout the program without further input from the user
Database	Software designed to store information in a systematic way, and at the same time to allow easy retrieval and manipulation of all data
Internet Access	**Attachment** A document sent with an e-mail. Attachments should not be opened if the sender is not known to the operator as they may contain viruses **Data compression** The reduction in size of information to decrease transferred film size **Digital bandwidth** The amount of information in bits per second (bps), kilobits per second (kbps), or megabits per second (Mbps) that can be sent via a communication channel or a network connection in a set period of time **Domain name** Locates an organisation or individual on the internet **e-mail** An electronic mail system. Its current uses include sending imaging reports and pathology reports directly to GP surgeries from one computer to another via Healthlink. It may also be used by GPs for the direct referral of patients for examinations **Internet** The worldwide network of computers **ISDN (Integrated Services Digital Network)** A set of standards for the transfer of digital information over a telephone wire and other media **ISP (Internet Service Provider)** A company that allows connection to the internet **MIME** (**M**ultipurpose **I**nternet **M**ail **E**xtensions) A method of sending binary objects by e-mail **POP (Post Office Protocol)** An e-mail system **WWW (World Wide Web)** An information and resource centre for the internet **Search engine** A database of key words that internet users can access to find information on the web **Server** A method of enabling computers to communicate with each other either by using another computer or software on a computer **Service provider** Organisations that offer connections to the internet

(continued on next page)

TYPES OF SOFTWARE *continued*

Internet Access *(contd)*	**Spam** Unrequested e-mail – usually advertising products or services **SSL (Secure Socket Layer)** A method of verifying the identity of system users and websites **URL (Uniform Resource Locator)** The address of internet files
Programming	**Address** A number which designates a particular storage area in the memory of the computer **Algorithm** Logical steps which define how a problem can be solved **BASIC (Beginners All-purpose Symbolic Instruction Code)** A high level language for computers and almost universally used for home computers **Editing** Altering the text or program **Flowchart** A diagrammatic representation of a computer program **FORTRAN** A programming language which is between BASIC and machine code in difficulty **Heuristic** A 'trial and error' method of trying to solve a problem **Initialise** At the beginning of computation all variables are given specific values in the program, e.g. A = 1, B = 7, C = 4, in this example, A, B and C are the variables initialised at those values **Iteration** To repeatedly execute an instruction in a program, e.g. 100 FOR X = 1 TO 200: NEXT X • In line 100, the routine has been iterated (repeated) 200 times **Java** A programming language that works on all computer systems **LISP (LISt Processor language)** A high level language used in Artificial Intelligence research **LOGO** A high level language usually used in schools to introduce primary school children to computers **Menu** A set of choices presented in a program, e.g.: 1. New patient 2. Alter patient details 3. Next appointment 4. Report details ENTER NUMBER OF CHOICE **Output** Data and information leaving a computer. This data can then be sent to a display screen, printer or another computer **PASCAL** A high level language for computers **Program** A set of written instructions for the computer

(continued on next page)

TYPES OF SOFTWARE *continued*

Programming (*contd*)	**PROM** (**P**rogrammable **R**ead **O**nly **M**emory) A specially-prepared chip which can be programmed, turning it into a Read Only Memory **Protocol** Written standards for the transfer of information between different computers **Real time** Usually defined as a computer controlling, or recording, events as they are actually happening **Remark (REM)** This instruction is ignored by the computer, but enables the user to add comments in plain English **ROM** (**R**ead **O**nly **M**emory) The pre-programmed part of the computer which enables it to run programs. While it may be accessible to the user, it cannot be altered **Statement** An instruction in a program **Subroutine** A self-contained part of a program which can be returned to time and time again within a program **Syntax error** Two words which are shown on the display when an incorrect input or statement has been made **Turnkey** A term used to denote a company which will provide all the necessary software and hardware plus back-up support to enable the user to '*turn a key*' and use the equipment **Zap** A small alteration to a program
Security	**Bug** A problem in the computer or (usually) in the program **Debugging** The finding and correction of errors or bugs in a program **Dongle** Any device used to protect software from piracy **Encryption** A method of coding data to prevent unauthorised access to the information **Firewall** A security system to prevent unauthorised access to information **Passwords** Entry is forbidden into many computer controlled systems unless a particular password has been entered. This provides fairly good security and virtually stops unwarranted interference with the data. Passwords are frequently graded, so that limited access to the system is allowed by some passwords but unlimited access is provided by other passwords **Time bomb** A device used by some software suppliers to prevent piracy of programmes. The software is protected by a certain phrase or code which can be removed by the legitimate supplier; if it is not removed the software is so arranged that it will wipe itself out after a period of use and erase all records **Virus** A program introduced into the computer system to corrupt the main program. New disks should always be checked before being used in the hospital computer system
Legal Issues	**Data Protection Act** Only registered users can hold information about individuals on computer and all patients have a right under this act to see any records concerning themselves or their treatment

THE ADVANTAGES OF COMPUTERISATION	
Eliminates Repetitive Tasks	• Repetitive form-filling not required • Once a patient's name has been entered, it should not have to be re-entered
Eliminates Paper Handling and Filing	Elimination of hardcopies of: • Request forms • Reports • Films • Paper records • Referral letters
Improves Inter-departmental Communications	Virtually instant access to: • Existing patient records films/images • Previous reports • New images and reports • Laboratory tests and results • Referral letters
Improves efficiency	Elimination of: • Manual filing of films/images • Manual retrieval of films/images • Need to copy images • Need to file images separate from patient records
Improves Confidentiality and Security	• Files, reports and patient details can be very secure • Passwords would only allow access to specific levels of information
Automated Data Collection	Improves information handling on, e.g.: • Staffing • Budgeting • Patient attendances • Use of equipment • Servicing • Research

THE PATIENT JOURNEY	

Overview	• Examination request is made, including clinical details
	• The request is accepted (or rejected)
	• The appointment is made
	• Instructions and information sent to the patient
	• DICOM worklist is generated
	• The examination is completed and it is electronically signed that the work has been done
	• Images sent to PACS
	• PACS acknowledgement of receipt of the images
	• Additional examinations/images added to file using PACS and DICOM
	• The image, notes and clinical details placed on PACS workstation
	• Image is reported on using voice recognition software
	• The report is electronically signed
	• Text is automatically available on:
	  ○ Radiological Information System (RIS)
	  ○ Hospital Information System (HIS)
	  ○ Electronic Patient Record (EPR)

Integrating Health Enterprise (IHE)	An initiative introduced in 1999 **Aim:** • To bring together manufacturers of clinical information systems, PACS systems and imaging equipment • To talk about integration requirements and systems

(continued on next page)

THE PATIENT JOURNEY *continued*	

Individual Computer Systems	**Overview**
	• The hospital information system (HIS) is the central hub
	• Other systems are linked to it, e.g.
	  ◦ Picture Archiving and Communication Systems (PACS)
	  ◦ Electronic Patient Record (EPR)
	  ◦ Electronic Remote Requesting System (RRS)
	  ◦ Radiological Information System (RIS)
	• DICOM is the protocol used so that the different parts can communicate with each other
	
	Fig. 4.1 Individual computer systems.

Web-based Integration	Works in a similar way to the World Wide Web and has: • An internet server • A search engine • Stores information on the web • RIS and HIS, etc. are stored as data sets • User can browse the individual data sets **Advantages** • Upgrades can be done on the central server • Navigation is done using a mouse • Hyperlinks can be used to aid the search facility
Digital Imaging and Communications in Medicine (DICOM)	An initiative sponsored by the Radiological Society of North America and the Health and Management Systems Society **Aim** • To integrate information and management systems so that clinical information can be communicated among all specialities and providers • Any doctor will eventually have access to a wide range of tests and images, on computer • The primary concern is patient confidentiality • Now accepted worldwide in the imaging field (See DICOM p. 3)
Health Level 7 (HL7)	• A standard less well designed than DICOM • Used for HIS and RIS systems • Originally used by North American manufacturers • HL7 and DICOM equipment can be integrated together
Picture Archiving and Communication Systems (PACS)	• PACS is a method of storing images in a digital format • Once stored, they can be sent to different parts of the hospital and to the wider medical community. • (See PACS p. 59)

Electronic Patient Record (EPR)	**Aims to contain**
	• Individual details:
	  ◦ Patient name
	  ◦ Address
	  ◦ Date of birth
	  ◦ Hospital number

(continued on next page)

THE PATIENT JOURNEY *continued*

Electronic Patient Record (EPR) *(contd)*	○ NHS number ○ Next of kin, etc. • Includes: ○ Hospital records ○ GP records ○ Discharge summaries ○ Clinical letters ○ Prescribing data • Information added to the record is automatically added to the other systems (e.g. HIS, PACS, RIS)
Hospital Information System (HIS)	• A computerised system, the aim of which it to build a network of complementary centres, e.g. ○ Hospitals ○ Laboratories ○ Primary Care Trusts and ○ GP centres, etc. spread throughout Europe • To meet the social and healthcare needs in each area • The term can also be used to define the system used in an individual hospital or unit **Aims to contain all patient information, e.g.** • Individual details: ○ Patient name ○ Address ○ Date of birth ○ Hospital number ○ NHS number ○ General Practitioner ○ Next of kin, etc. • Reports from clinical investigations, e.g. ○ Imaging ○ Bronchoscopic investigations ○ Endoscopy ○ Tissue cultures, etc. • Laboratory test results ○ Biochemistry ○ Bacteriology ○ Haematology ○ Immunology ○ Virology, etc. • Additional information ○ Hospital admissions ○ Out patient appointments ○ Discharge information • Information added to the record is automatically added to the other systems (e.g. EPR, PACS, RIS) • Only a limited number of people can input data to ensure accuracy of the information held
Electronic Remote Requesting System (RRS))	• A method of electronically requesting tests and examinations from: ○ Hospital wards ○ Out-patient clinics ○ GP surgeries
Order Communications (OCM)	• Each department being accessed requires a standardised request form on the system, e.g. ○ Imaging ○ Haematology ○ Pathology, etc. **Structure** • A module of HIS • Must be integrated with RIS to be able to access:

(continued on next page)

THE PATIENT JOURNEY *continued*

Order Communications (OCM) (*contd*)	○ Previous imaging procedures ○ Previous reports ○ Room availability and booking • Must be integrated with PACS to allow: ○ Clinical reports and images to appear on the diagnostic workstations **Advantages** • Electronic generic request forms • Patient information can be obtained from HIS • Elimination of paper request forms • Reports have only to be entered once • Digital signing of forms using a code for patient security **Disadvantages** • If standardised lists are used, e.g. reasons for imaging requests, the exact reason may not be on the list • Digital codes can be passed on to unauthorised users

Radiological Information System (RIS)	• RIS is a text-based computer system for:
	  ○ Booking appointments
	  ○ Allocating rooms
	  ○ Storing reports
	  ○ Auditing workflow of all staff
	
	Using the system
	• Request for examination is received
	• User logs on – so that a record is kept of the people using the system
	• HIS is checked to see if the patient is on the system
	• Note systems advise if a duplicate entry is suspected
	• An RIS number is allocated
	• If not on the system (if they have not attended the hospital before as an in-patient or out-patient) an RIS number is allocated
	• If the patient details are not known, a local protocol needs to be in place to allocate an RIS number, e.g.
	  ○ If the patient is unconscious
	  ○ Protocols could include a date of birth of 30 February, etc.
	• If the patient information requires changing on HIS (e.g. a change of address), on modern systems this can be done from RIS
	• A worklist is generated
	• When integrated with PACS the reports can be added to the images
	
	Imaging the patient
	• The operator logs on
	• The patient details are checked
	• The order is modified if necessary, e.g.
	  ○ Adding additional examinations
	  ○ Changing incorrect requests, e.g. right for left
	• The patient is imaged
	• The patient leaves
	• The operator records:
	  ○ The name of the person undertaking the examination
	  ○ The room used
	  ○ Size and number of films taken
	  ○ Exposure details
	  ○ Comments
	• The operator logs off

(continued on next page)

THE PATIENT JOURNEY *continued*

| **Radiological Information System (RIS)** (*contd*) | **Reporting**
• The images are viewed on a workstation
• Previous images can be viewed alongside
• Voice activated software can be used for reporting
• The report can be stored on RIS
• The report and images can be available on PACS

Auditing
The system can be used for auditing and creating management reports, e.g.
• Staffing
• Room usage
• Budgeting
• Patient attendances
• Time taken for examinations
• Use of equipment
• Ordering information

Links to conventional film filing system
• Can be used as a database for the conventional system by logging:
 ○ When a film is removed
 ○ The date and time it is removed
 ○ The name of the person requesting the film file
 ○ Date and time of its return
• It can also be interrogated to identify:
 ○ Who last requested a film file
 ○ When they requested it
• Automatically generate letters requesting the return after a set length of time
• Clinics can generate requests for film files prior to appointments
• Ideally HIS would automatically request film files prior to clinics to allow for the files to be obtained |

TERMINOLOGY	
Aspect Ratio	The ratio of the width of a display screen to the height, e.g. 4:3
Bezel	The plastic or metal frame round a display screen
Brightness (Luminance)	The amount of light a LCD monitor produces in candela (cd) per square metre (m^2), e.g. 250 to 350 cd/m^2
Colour Depth	The number of bits used to give the colour of one pixel, and gives the number of different colours that can be displayed at one time, e.g. • 1 bit depth gives 2 colours (black and white) • 16 bit depth gives 65563 colours that can be displayed • 24 bit depth gives 16.8 million colours that can be displayed
Contrast Ratio	The difference in intensity between the black and white on an LCD screen • The higher the contrast ratio the better the detail
Cursor	A flashing marker on the screen which indicates where the next character is to be inserted
Dot Pitch	A measure of the sharpness or resolution of a screen • DPM – dots per millimetre • The higher the figure the better the resolution of the screen as the dots are closer together
LCD	Liquid Crystal Display monitor
Monitor	A device very similar to a television, but which receives video signals directly from the computer
Native Resolution	The optimum resolution of a LCD monitor. If this is changed the image quality diminishes Examples of native resolution: • 17 inch screen = 1024 × 768 • 20 inch screen = 1600 × 1200
Pixel	Picture cell. A pixel is the smallest number of dots which can be used by a character on the display screen
Refresh Rate	Number of times the monitor is scanned by the electron beam per second • The higher the refresh rate the less screen flicker • A refresh rate of 85 Hertz means the screen is scanned 85 times each second
Resolution	The number of 'dots' on a monitor screen defines the resolution of a system by describing the number of pixels horizontally and vertically, e.g. 1200 × 1200 gives a resolution of 1200 separate points horizontally and vertically
RGB Input	The colour input on a monitor. The signal from the computer is taken by the monitor as a basic **R**ed, **G**reen and **B**lue input
Screen Size	Cathode ray tubes • The diagonal measurement from the outer corners of the casing Liquid Crystal Display screens • The diagonal measurement from the corners of the screen
Scrolling	The movement of text or data on the display screen. Scrolling can be upwards, downwards or sideways
Thermionic Emission	The release of electrons when a substance is heated

(continued on next page)

TERMINOLOGY *continued*	
VDU	Visual display unit
Viewing Angle	The maximum horizontal and vertical angle that a monitor screen can be viewed at to give a clear image with accurate colours, e.g. • 120° • 170°
Voxel	A three-dimensional pixel
Interlacing	Consider one still picture on a cathode ray monitor (Figs 5.1, 5.2) • The picture is made up of two fields which consist, in a 625 line system, of 312.5 lines each • Each horizontal line is made up of minute dots (pixels) • The picture is constructed by an electron beam scanning the tube phosphor from top left to bottom right in a series of horizontal lines • First the odd lines are scanned, the beam jumps back to the top left and then the even lines are scanned • This system of constructing the frame is called 'double interlacing' • ×4 and ×8 interlacing will produce images which, are virtually line free 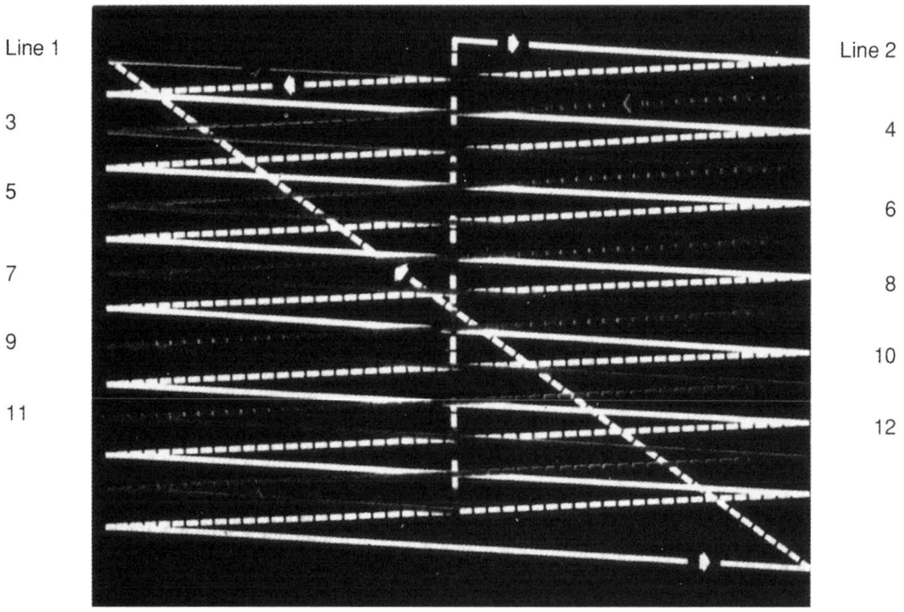

Fig. 5.1 Odd, then even lines are scanned.

(continued on next page)

Interlacing (*contd*)

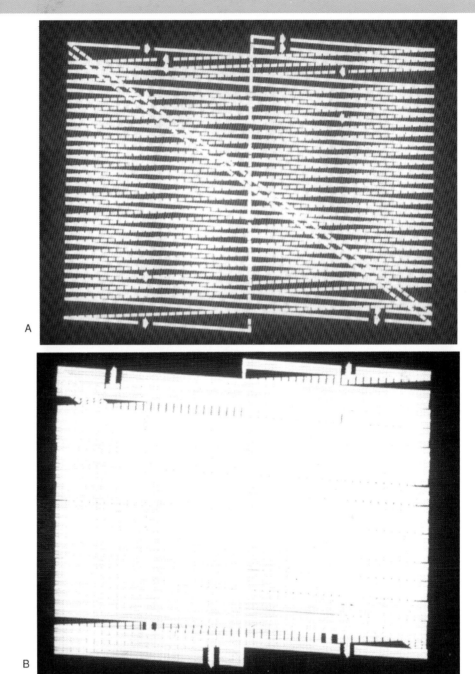

Fig. 5.2 Multiple interlacing. (A) ×2 Interlacing. (B) Raster lines almost disappear.

VISUAL DISPLAY EQUIPMENT

Principle of Operation	• Electricity can either be on or off • The signal is received by the visual display unit in the form of a stream of electrons (on) and gaps (off) • The stream of electrons and gaps scan across the screen from side to side, slowly moving down (see interlacing) • When an electron hits a pixel on the screen the pixel lights up • When a 'gap' is present the pixel does not light • Therefore a black and white image is formed on the screen

Cathode Ray Tubes	Composed of:
	• A negative cathode
	  ○ When heated produces a stream of electrons by thermionic emission
	• A grid
	  ○ To focus the electron beam
	• A positive anode
	  ○ Attracts the electron beam from the cathode
	• Deflecting coils
	  ○ Focus the electron beam
	  ○ Move the beam across the fluorescent screen from side to side
	• A fluorescent screen
	  ○ Coated with phosphors which have a characteristic light emission
	  ○ The phosphors are given numbers, e.g.
	    – P45, P4 and P40 emit white light (a mixture of blue and green)
	    – P11 emits blue light
	    – P31 and P24 emit green light
	
	In colour monitors:
	• Red, green and blue emitting phosphors are used
	• Phosphors are arranged in groups of either dots or strips
	• A shadow mask
	  ○ A perforated metal plate next to the fluorescent screen
	  ○ Allows accurate focusing of the electron beam
	  ○ The perforations match the phosphor dots
	• An aperture grill
	  ○ Strips of wire
	  ○ Allows accurate focusing of the electron beam
	  ○ The gaps between the wires match the phosphor strips
	• A slot mask
	  ○ Combines a shadow mask and an aperture grill
	  ○ Uses vertical slots
	  ○ Creates a brighter image

FLAT SCREEN MONITORS

Gas Plasma Monitors	**Construction**
	• Front glass plate
	  ○ Protects and supports the screen
	• Display electrode
	  ○ Arranged in horizontal rows
	• Dielectric layer
	  ○ Provides insulation
	• Magnesium oxide layer
	  ○ Protective layer
	• Pixel layer
	  ○ Each pixel contains neon gas and is placed between two electrodes
	  ○ Each pixel made of three sub pixels – green, red and blue
	  ○ By varying the current pulse different combinations can be illuminated

(continued on next page)

FLAT SCREEN MONITORS *continued*

Gas Plasma Monitors (contd)	• Phosphor ○ Coated on the inside of each pixel cell • Address electrode ○ Arranged in vertical columns ○ Form a grid pattern with the display electrodes • Address protective layer ○ Protects electrodes • Rear glass plate ○ Supports and protects the screen **Principles of operation** • The computer charges the electrodes at the point where they cross • An electric current is formed in the pixel gas at that point • The charged particles in the gas cause the release of ultraviolet photons • The photons react with the phosphor coating causing an electron to be raised to a higher energy level • When the electron returns to its normal energy band it releases a visible light photon • The image can then be viewed on the monitor • By varying the current from the computer the brightness and colour combination of the image can be varied
Liquid Crystal Displays (Active)	**Construction** • Backlight ○ Illuminates the substrate • Substrate ○ Polarised glass • Liquid crystal material ○ Forms a thin layer trapped between the substrate • Thin film transistor (TFT) ○ A matrix of transistors and capacitors • Substrate ○ Polarised glass **Principles of operation** • Works by blocking light • The rear substrate is back lit • The computer sends a signal to a specific pixel ○ In the TFT the specific row is switched on and a charge is sent down the specific column ○ The capacitor aligned to the pixel receives a charge ○ The charge causes the liquid crystal molecules to block some of the light ○ This gives the colour and image on the second substrate • The capacitor remains charged until the next refresh cycle
Liquid Crystal Displays (Passive)	• Work as active LCD • Grid of conductive metal replaces TFT • Rarely used due to: ○ Slow response times ○ Poor voltage control

LASERS

Light and the Laser	**White light**

White light
- Made up of varying wavelengths
- Ranges from ultraviolet in the short wave, through visible light, to infrared in the long wavelengths
- Very short coherence lengths, due to the number of different wavelengths and the anti-phase components cancelling one another out

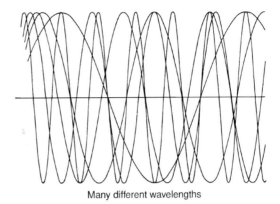

Many different wavelengths

Fig. 6.1 White light – a cacophony in vision.

Laser light
- Only one wavelength

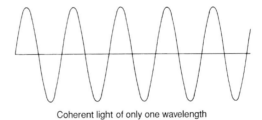

Coherent light of only one wavelength

Fig. 6.2 Laser light – coherent light of only one wavelength.

The First Laser

Pulsed laser
In 1960, Theodore Maiman, working at the Hughes Aircraft Electronic Research Laboratory, built the first laser
- It was basically a photographer's electronic flashgun wound around a crystal of synthetic ruby (aluminium oxide mixed with a small amount of chromium)
- The synthetic ruby was in the form of a tube with a mirror at each end of the tube
- One mirror was a partial reflector
- The distance between the mirrors was precisely defined
- It was tuned to make the light produced bounce back and forth in a regular and reinforcing pattern to create standing waves of light in the rod which had a pulse of about three thousandths of a second

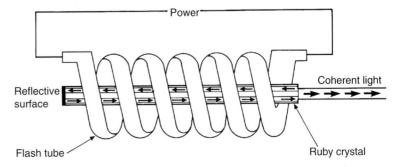

Fig. 6.3 Maiman's original synthetic ruby laser.

THE OPERATION OF A LASER

The Basic Physics	• If a photon is fired at an atom, the atom can absorb the photon and thus be raised to an excited state
	• The only way that the atom can return to stability is by releasing this absorbed energy in the form of a photon of light (*spontaneous emission*)
	• But if a photon is fired at an already excited atom, the atom will release TWO light photons and then return to its stable state (*stimulated emission*) (Fig. 6.4)

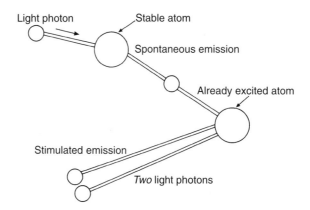

Fig. 6.4 Stimulated emission.

Inside a Laser	• The atoms are stimulated by an external power source to produce stimulated emission
	• When a stage is reached, whereby half the atoms are in an excited state, *population inversion* occurs (Fig. 6.5)
	• If more photons are then fired, *stimulated emission* takes place. Stimulated emission occurs because it is more likely that the photons will strike an already excited atom rather than a stable atom
	• If the above events occur in a tube, the tube can be 'tuned' to encourage the light produced to oscillate in a regular pattern
	• The light then breaks out as an extremely coherent, parallel beam of light which contains a considerable amount of energy – laser light

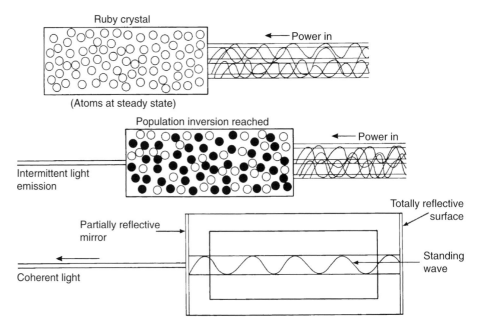

Fig. 6.5 Population inversion.

(continued on next page)

THE OPERATION OF A LASER *continued*

Continuous Wave Gas Laser	• Uses helium and neon as the lasing material • The light is very coherent and uniform and can be switched off and on like an electric light • They are used in laser imagers 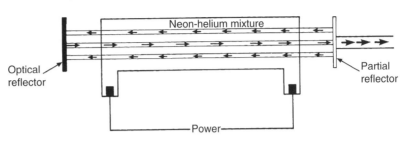 **Fig. 6.6** Continuous wave gas laser.

THE ORIGINAL LASER IMAGERS

	Fig. 6.7 Principles of a laser imager.
Operator Keypad	This allows control of the parameters for imaging at the time of the examination These can include: • Film size • Format, i.e. the number of images recorded on the film • Image-store sequence • Density • Contrast • Exposure • Image polarity • Clear or black border background • Number of copies required • Patient information • Automatic hospital name, date recording • Printing of the image
Exposure	The patient is imaged
Memory Store	All the digital image information required for one 'film' must be put into the memory store, before the image recording can start • The image is stored in the RAM memory of the unit which has a basic memory capable of storing information to fill one 35×43 cm film from each modality at a time • When the memory is full, a film is automatically dispensed (by either gravity or rollers) and is positioned ready for scanning
An Interface	Transmits the digital information from the memory store to the laser

(continued on next page)

THE ORIGINAL LASER IMAGERS *continued*	
An Acoustic-optical Modulator	Modulates the laser beam in terms of brightness, grey levels, etc.
The Laser	• Lasers produce coherent beams of parallel light and therefore the scanning optics can be much simpler than if white light is used, which produces a divergent beam • Either a red, helium-neon laser, which emits light of 632 nm, or an infrared laser in the range of 750–850 nm, can be used • The information from the memory store is used to modulate the laser beam in terms of brightness, grey scales, etc. and therefore the intensity of the beam will be determined by the digital value of the input signal
An Optical System	A lens system is used to focus the laser beam onto a scanner
A (Mechanical) Scanner	A very accurate and fast Galvano scanner used to move the laser beam from side to side across the imaging field
A Mirror	**Horizontal scanning** • The beam is focused using an optical lens system onto a moving mirror system which moves the beam from side to side across the film, printing one line of information at a time • Each line is capable of containing between 3500 and 4100 pixels of information
A (Mechanical) Film Transport System	**Vertical imaging** • After each line has been printed, the film moves vertically down to allow the next line to be printed • Each film will have to move between 4250 and 5100 times before imaging has been completed
Imaging	Takes between 8 and 30 seconds
Film Characteristics	• The film is 'written on' by the laser, therefore only a single-sided, fine grain, silver halide emulsion is required • This is mounted on either a blue tinted or a clear polyester base with an antihalation layer to prevent curl **Note** It is important that the correct film is purchased to match the type of laser used to obtain optimum results • *Helium-neon lasers* produce red light and therefore the film should have a sensitivity in the order of 633 nm and special green safelight filters may be purchased if required for darkroom film handling • *Infrared lasers* require film with a sensitivity of between 780 and 850 nm and should be handled in total darkness
Processing	• The film is packaged so that it can be loaded into the laser printer in daylight conditions and, from the printer, it is automatically fed into the automatic processing unit • Or, into a light-proof receiving magazine which is closed and taken to a separate automatic processor
Digital Input Signal	• Can either be transferred directly to the printer from the separate modalities • Or can be stored on computer disk and then taken to the laser imager • Or can be digitally stored and viewed only on a computer It is possible for the imagers to receive input signals at the same time as they are 'writing' an image and therefore there is no processing delay

IMAGING PLATES

| Imaging Plate Construction | 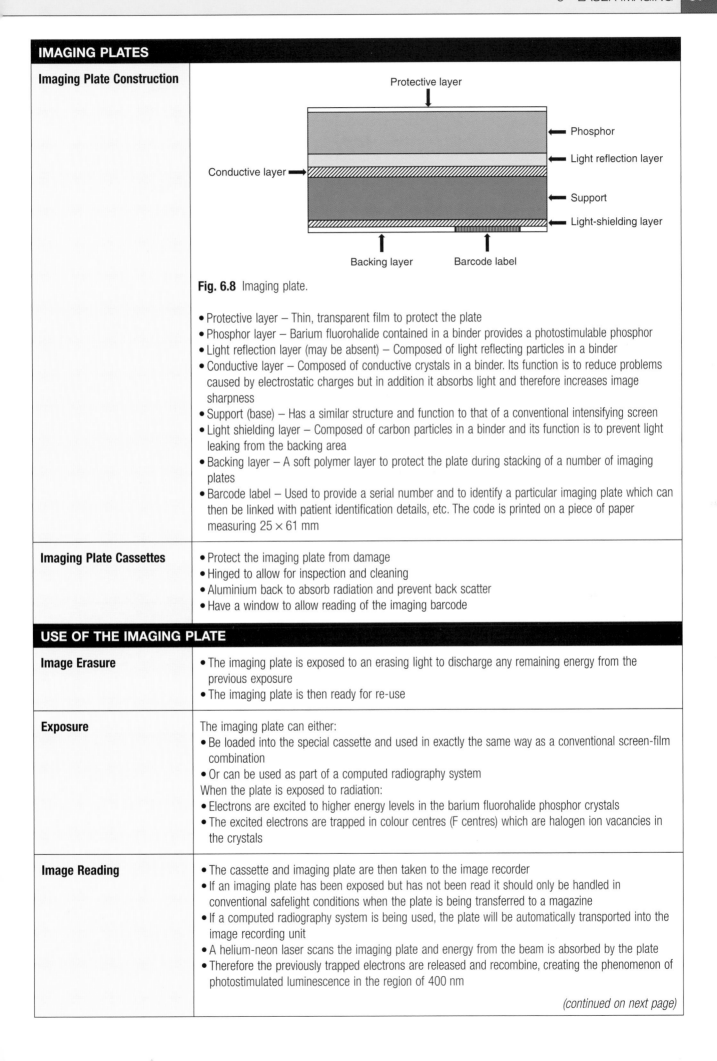 |

Fig. 6.8 Imaging plate.

- Protective layer – Thin, transparent film to protect the plate
- Phosphor layer – Barium fluorohalide contained in a binder provides a photostimulable phosphor
- Light reflection layer (may be absent) – Composed of light reflecting particles in a binder
- Conductive layer – Composed of conductive crystals in a binder. Its function is to reduce problems caused by electrostatic charges but in addition it absorbs light and therefore increases image sharpness
- Support (base) – Has a similar structure and function to that of a conventional intensifying screen
- Light shielding layer – Composed of carbon particles in a binder and its function is to prevent light leaking from the backing area
- Backing layer – A soft polymer layer to protect the plate during stacking of a number of imaging plates
- Barcode label – Used to provide a serial number and to identify a particular imaging plate which can then be linked with patient identification details, etc. The code is printed on a piece of paper measuring 25×61 mm

| Imaging Plate Cassettes | - Protect the imaging plate from damage
- Hinged to allow for inspection and cleaning
- Aluminium back to absorb radiation and prevent back scatter
- Have a window to allow reading of the imaging barcode |

USE OF THE IMAGING PLATE

| Image Erasure | - The imaging plate is exposed to an erasing light to discharge any remaining energy from the previous exposure
- The imaging plate is then ready for re-use |

| Exposure | The imaging plate can either:
- Be loaded into the special cassette and used in exactly the same way as a conventional screen-film combination
- Or can be used as part of a computed radiography system
When the plate is exposed to radiation:
- Electrons are excited to higher energy levels in the barium fluorohalide phosphor crystals
- The excited electrons are trapped in colour centres (F centres) which are halogen ion vacancies in the crystals |

| Image Reading | - The cassette and imaging plate are then taken to the image recorder
- If an imaging plate has been exposed but has not been read it should only be handled in conventional safelight conditions when the plate is being transferred to a magazine
- If a computed radiography system is being used, the plate will be automatically transported into the image recording unit
- A helium-neon laser scans the imaging plate and energy from the beam is absorbed by the plate
- Therefore the previously trapped electrons are released and recombine, creating the phenomenon of photostimulated luminescence in the region of 400 nm |

(continued on next page)

USE OF THE IMAGING PLATE *continued*

Image Reading (*contd*)	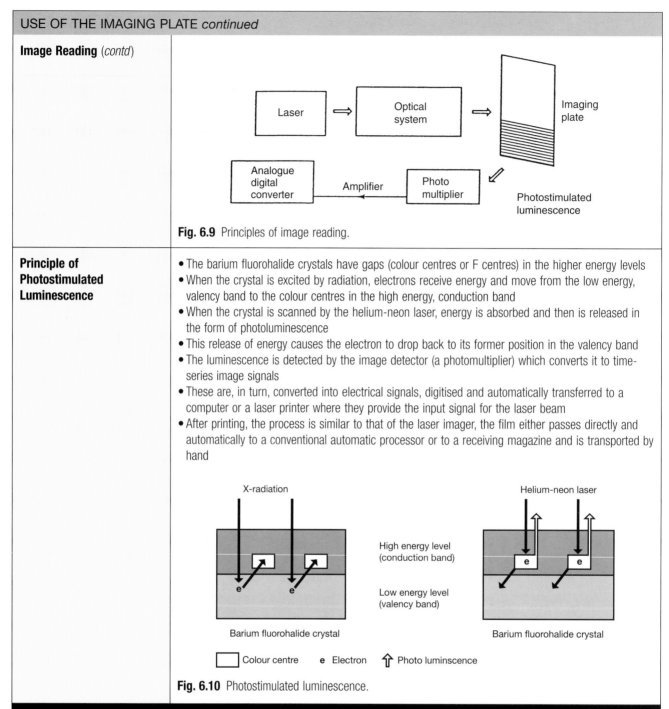

Fig. 6.9 Principles of image reading.

Principle of Photostimulated Luminescence

- The barium fluorohalide crystals have gaps (colour centres or F centres) in the higher energy levels
- When the crystal is excited by radiation, electrons receive energy and move from the low energy, valency band to the colour centres in the high energy, conduction band
- When the crystal is scanned by the helium-neon laser, energy is absorbed and then is released in the form of photoluminescence
- This release of energy causes the electron to drop back to its former position in the valency band
- The luminescence is detected by the image detector (a photomultiplier) which converts it to time-series image signals
- These are, in turn, converted into electrical signals, digitised and automatically transferred to a computer or a laser printer where they provide the input signal for the laser beam
- After printing, the process is similar to that of the laser imager, the film either passes directly and automatically to a conventional automatic processor or to a receiving magazine and is transported by hand

Fig. 6.10 Photostimulated luminescence.

DRY FILM PROCESSING

Technology is available which utilises direct laser printing to produce an image without the use of processing chemicals

Film Characteristics

- The 12 × 24 cm film can be handled in daylight conditions and is either a blue or clear polyester-based film with a carbon coating
- The carbon responds digitally to laser energy over a certain threshold value
- Each pixel on the film contains in excess of 4000 sub-pixel elements called pels. The whole film has a scratch resistant 'overcoat'

Imaging

- The digital signal from the appropriate modality is fed into solid state laser diodes which then scan the film in a way similar to that of other laser printers
- As the signal is digital the pels are either exposed or not exposed and because of their very small size and large numbers shades of grey can be built up as a result
- The film is ready for viewing in 90 seconds

(continued on next page)

DRY FILM PROCESSING *continued*

Imaging System Characteristics	• Resolution of 4000 × 5000 pixels, with 256 grey levels • Transfer of data is in the order of 8–30 seconds • The image can be manipulated and the parameters changed prior to printing • The laser imager is very susceptible to dust and vibration, particularly when the laser beam transfer is via a mirror • Any vertical movement of the film by mechanical means must remain absolutely in register throughout the whole of the exposure. Any interruption of this travel, caused by vibration or mechanical movement, will produce gross artefacts on the image • As the optics for laser imagers are fairly simple there tends to be little image distortion

AIM OF IMAGE MANIPULATION	
	To produce an excellent image to maximise diagnostic accuracy

TERMINOLOGY	
Analogue	Represents a quantity changing in steps which are continuous, i.e. a sine wave
Brightness	The intensity values of the individual pixels in an image, the lower the brightness the darker the image
Compression	The reduction in size (in bytes) of an image to save storage space
Contrast	The density difference between two adjacent areas on the image
Digital	An image comprised of discrete areas or pixels
Edge Enhancement	The highlighting of a straight line or edge of an object to visually increase the sharpness of the image
Fourier Transform	A method of mathematically changing data, e.g. changing spatial data to frequency data
Frequency Data	The number of times a specific value occurs in an image
Heuristic	When an image is automatically improved because the program has changed due to a previous imaging experience
Hough Transform	A method of highlighting areas of a specific shape within an image
Noise	Anything that may detract from the image
Resolution (Sharpness)	The size of the smallest object or distance between two objects that must exist before the imaging system will record that object or objects as separate entities.
Segmentation	Selection of an area of interest and eliminating unwanted data. Can be done manually or automatically with an appropriate software package
Signal	The information required from the imaging system, e.g. the radiograph, the minimum size of the object that must be visible
Spatial Data	Gives the position of the varying intensities (brightness) across an image
Spatial Frequency	Object size, measured in line pairs per millimetre
Spatial Resolution	The smallest part of an image that can be seen
Window	The range of colour (or grey) scale values displayed on a digital image

DIGITISING AN ANALOGUE IMAGE	
An Analogue Image	• Two dimensional image • Different shades of grey • The shading is continuous throughout the image
A Digital Image	• Two dimensional image • Different shades of grey (or colours – red, green blue) • The grey is made up of discrete areas or pixels
Changing an Analogue Image to a Digital Image	• Take the analogue image • Imagine a grid superimposed over the image – usually 512 × 512 or 1024 × 1024 • The brightness (amount of grey) in each square (pixel) in the image is measured

(continued on next page)

DIGITISING AN ANALOGUE IMAGE *continued*	
Changing an Analogue Image to a Digital Image (*contd*)	• Each pixel can then be given a number representing the brightness/shade of grey • Usually each pixel is given a value between 0 and 256 • This gives the image numerical values, i.e. digitises it
Nyquist Theorem	States that an analogue signal waveform may be reconstructed without error from a sample which is equal to, or greater than, twice the highest frequency in the analogue signal, e.g. • To digitally convert a 2 MHz signal, a sample must be taken at 4 MHz • To give a resolution of 5 line pairs per millimeter, each line pair equals 0.2 mm therefore a pixel sample must be measured at 0.1 mm intervals
Fourier Transform	• A method of mathematically changing data, e.g. changing spatial data to frequency data • Spatial data give the position of the varying intensities (brightness) across an image

IMAGE ENHANCEMENT

	Methods of manipulating the pixel values to improve or enhance the area of interest in the image
Windowing	• Process of using the pixels to make an image • 256 shades of grey are usually assigned • But the human eye can only determine about 100 shades of grey • The shades of grey can be distributed over a wide or a narrow range of pixels
Narrow Window	• The grey is distributed over a narrow range of units • The central unit is the average pixel number for the structure of interest • If the average pixel was 50 and a narrow window of 170 was selected, then pixels of 85 (half 170) above and below 50 would be used • Therefore the grey scale would extend from −35 to 135 • Any readings below −35 would be pure black • Any readings above 135 would be pure white
Wide Window	• The grey is distributed over a wide range of pixels • The central unit is the average pixel number for the structure of interest • If the average pixel was 400 and a wide window of 2000 was selected, then pixels of 1000 (half 2000) above and below 400 would be used • Therefore the grey scale would extend from − 600 to 1400 • Any readings below − 600 would be pure black • Any readings above 1400 would be pure white

ADJUSTING NOISE AND CONTRAST

Signal to Noise Ratio	Image quality may be defined as the signal to noise ratio: $$\text{Image quality} = \frac{\text{signal}}{\text{noise}}$$ The signal is the information required from the imaging system • The signal can be defined as the minimum size of the object that must be visible The noise is anything that may detract from that signal • The noise, on the monitor, could be defined as the graininess of the image
Image Quality	• If the sharpness of the system is increased, the visually disturbing noise will also increase, as now the system is resolving the noise better as well as giving a sharper signal • If the contrast is increased the signal will appear to be clearer, but so will the noise • To compensate for all the factors is impossible, therefore the final result has to be a compromise (Fig. 7.1)

(continued on next page)

ADJUSTING NOISE AND CONTRAST *continued*

Image Quality (*contd*)	**Fig. 7.1** Image quality is a compromise between sharpness, contrast and noise.
Contrast	A radiograph is the product of a transfer of information. During this transfer it is exposed to a number of different influences. Contrast helps to determine the quality of the radiograph **There are three principal 'types' of contrast** • Subject contrast • Image contrast • Radiographic contrast
Subject Contrast	Subject contrast (Fig. 7.2) can be defined as the ratio of the emergent intensities, i.e.: $$\text{Subject contrast} = \frac{1_F}{1_B}$$ • This is caused by differential attenuation and absorption of the X-ray beam as it passes through the patient (i.e. the subject) • It is responsible for the differing intensities of the emergent X-ray beam, and therefore the exposures that eventually reach the film • Bone attenuates more of the beam than the fatty tissue and therefore the emergent intensity in the area below the bone is less than the surrounding fatty tissue • The film receives less exposure and produces a lower image density when compared to the fatty tissue areas $$\text{Subject contrast} = \frac{I_F}{I_B} \qquad \text{Radiographic contrast} = D_1 - D_2$$ **Fig. 7.2** Diagrammatic illustration of subject contrast.
Factors Affecting Subject Contrast	
Different Thicknesses of the Same Tissue Type	Subject contrast is the ratio of the intensity that has passed through the thin part, compared with the thicker part The thicker of the two will: • Attenuate more of the beam • Allow less exposure to reach the film

(continued on next page)

ADJUSTING NOISE AND CONTRAST *continued*

Different Densities of the Same Tissue with the Same Volume but at a Higher Density	Subject contrast is the ratio of the intensity that has passed through the less dense part, compared with the denser part The higher density will: • Attenuate more of the beam • Reduce the intensity of the emergent beam
Different Atomic Numbers of Different Tissues	The higher the atomic number: • The more the attenuation of the incident X-ray beam • The less the intensity of the emergent beam **Note** At the energies used in diagnostic radiography, photoelectric absorption predominates and is the largest contributing factor to subject contrast
Radiation Quality – The kiloVoltage (kV) Set for the Exposure	• Changing kV gives a high contrast variation in bone work • The influence of kV is smaller on soft tissue rendition • In the low kV range, 10 kV has more effect on contrast than in the higher kV range • In the middle kV range, 20 kV is needed to give an appreciable change in contrast For the same subject, increasing the kV: • Decreases the difference in intensities of the emergent beam • Therefore decreases the subject contrast Low kV will produce high subject contrast **Note** The kV must be high enough to adequately penetrate the area being examined
X-ray Equipment	Factors affecting subject contrast include: • The anode material, e.g. mammography • Varying voltage ripple components • Tube filters and supplementary filters
Scattered Radiation	Radiation fog, which increases the overall density of the image Scatter can be limited by: • Lowering the kV In general (below 150 kV), the lower the selected kV, the lower the amount of scatter and the lower the radiation fog and reduction in image latitude The use of: • Grids • Collimators
Use of Contrast Agents	Used to fill a cavity or space in the body that usually has a low subject contrast when compared with surrounding structures **Positive agents** • Non-ionic iodine compounds or barium which increase the X-ray absorption properties of the structure concerned **Negative agents** • Carbon dioxide or air which decrease the absorption properties, with an effect on the intensity of the emergent beam These can also be used in combination, e.g. double contrast barium meals and enemas
Radiographic Contrast	• This is the density difference between two adjacent areas on the image • These differences in density may or may not be observable to the naked eye
Subjective Contrast	• The eye analyses the structures in the radiograph and will select details • The success rate depends on the different degrees of brightness: ○ Density detail – Density surroundings • This variable indicates the difference in logarithmic form which suits the physiology of the eye *(continued on next page)*

ADJUSTING NOISE AND CONTRAST *continued*

Subjective Contrast (*contd*)	• This measurement is also the measurement of subjective contrast, i.e.
	  ○ Contrast = Density detail − Density surroundings
	• It is the observer's opinion of the contrast that is seen on the film
	• It is a combination of all the other factors listed, plus:
	  ○ Viewing conditions
	  ○ The performance of the eye
	  ○ The observers ability and perhaps their personal opinion

CONTRAST ENHANCEMENT IN DIGITAL IMAGING

Histogram Production	For a given image, a histogram can be produced, plotting: • Intensity level of the image pixels (horizontal axis) • Number of pixels (vertical axis)
Histogram Equalisation Software	• Alters a computer image to equally distribute the brightness levels over the whole histogram • This effect increases the contrast of the image **Note** If the intensity range of the original histogram is small the changed image will have a lot of noise • Used to lighten a dark image
Contrast Stretching Software	• If the image has a narrow range of intensity values the histogram can be 'stretched' to cover a specified upper and lower intensity range • This improves the contrast of the image without changing the range of grey levels

NOISE REDUCTION

Density Slicing or Thresholding	The separating (segmenting) of an area of interest and removing unwanted information. Works best if there is a clear peak on the histogram that can be selected
	• Either by selecting pixels of similar values (intensity threshold)
	  ○ The image is scanned
	  ○ Each pixel is compared with the threshold
	  ○ Those above the threshold are turned white
	  ○ Those below are turned black (or vice versa)
	• Or by selecting specific colours or intensities in the image background, e.g.
	  ○ The background pixels could be selected and turned black
	  ○ The remaining pixels are unchanged

Image Smoothing	**Neighbourhood averaging (Gaussian smoothing)**
	• Either the average value of the pixels is calculated
	• Or an area of the image is selected, e.g. 3 pixels by 3 pixels
	• This would result in 9 pixels being selected
	• The average value of the pixels is calculated by:
	  ○ Multiplying by 1/9, and adding the results together to find the average pixel value
	  ○ The resultant pixels form the mask kernel or spatial filter
	  ○ The mask is applied to the whole image
	• This removes the higher frequencies from the image
	• The resultant image has lower contrast
	
	Median filtering
	• The median pixel value is selected for the mask
	  ○ This preserves the edges of the image
	  ○ The pixels with the extreme values are reduced
	• The resultant image has less noise

Hough Transform	A method of highlighting areas of a specific shape in an image • As curved lines are usually used, the technique is useful for highlighting specific anatomical areas • The transform identifies a number of pixels that form a curved line

(continued on next page)

NOISE REDUCTION *continued*	

Hough Transform (*contd*)	• The technique looks for pixels of similar value and:
	  ◦ Calculates the distance from the origin (the coordinates of the centre of a circle)
	  ◦ Calculates the angle from the origin using coordinates (or the radius in a circle)
	  ◦ Puts the calculated values into an equation
	• A mesh is created from the equation and overlaid on the image
	• At each point on the image a measurement is made and compared with the mesh
	• Mesh points with higher values than the image are overlaid on the image accentuating the area of interest
	
	Note
	This process does not work if the image has a lot of noise as clear edges of the object have to be identified

Unsharpness	Unsharpness on a radiograph – total image unsharpness is caused by the following three factors: • Movement of the object • The geometry of the radiation beam • The imaging system
Movement of the Object	**Calculating movement** • The object speed (*v*) in any direction other than perpendicular to the film plane, in mm • Multiplied by the exposure time (*t*) in seconds • Multiplied by the enlargement ratio, i.e. the focus film distance (ffd) divided by the focus object distance (fod). (about 10–20%, providing macro techniques are not used) $$U_m = v \times t \times \text{ffd/fod}$$

Movement Unsharpness	Movement unsharpness can be either voluntary or involuntary
	
	Voluntary movement
	• Controlled by asking the patient to hold their breath
	• By the use of immobilisation devices
	
	Involuntary movement
	• The movement of organs
	• The fluid in vessels which cannot be controlled by the patient
	
	Example:
	• If organ movement is about 5 mm and an exposure time of 0.2 s
	  ◦ The unsharpness = 1 mm
	• If the exposure time was reduced to 0.02 second
	  ◦ The unsharpness = 0.1 mm
	Therefore unsharpness would be improved by a factor of 10

Geometric Unsharpness	This is caused because the focal spot in the tube is not a point source • For a point source, the edges of an object will be recorded as sharp edges on the film • For an extended source, each edge of the object receives a ray as if it were two separate points, causing the penumbra effect, which produces unsharpness • If the focus–object distance is reduced, then the unsharpness is increased

(continued on next page)

NOISE REDUCTION *continued*

Geometric Unsharpness
(contd)
	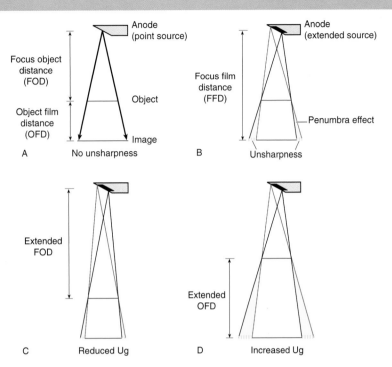
	
	Fig. 7.3 Effect of (A) point source, (B) extended source, (C) focus object distance and (D) object film distance on geometric unsharpness (Ug).
	
	Note
	• If the focus–object distance needs to be increased, to reduce geometric unsharpness, this will mean increasing the mAs and the exposure time, which increases movement unsharpness
	• If the object film distance (ofd) is increased geometric unsharpness is increased, and an increase in exposure will be required, which may increase movement unsharpness
	To calculate geometric unsharpness:
	• The ratio of the object film distance to the distance between the focal spot and the object is used
	• Therefore the larger the focal spot, the greater the distance between the object and the film, and the closer the focal spot is to the object, the more geometric unsharpness will increase
	
	Example
	If the focus film distance (ffd) = 100 cm and the focus object distance (fod) = 80 cm calculate the geometric unsharpness if a 1.2 mm focal spot was used
	• ofd = 100 − 80 = 20 cm
	  ○ geometric unsharpness:focal spot size = 20 : 80
	  ○ geometric unsharpness = $\frac{1}{4}$ of the focal spot size
	• If focal spot = 1.2 mm, then
	  ○ geometric unsharpness = $\frac{1.2}{4}$ = 0.3 mm

To Produce a Sharp Image	Theoretically use: • The shortest possible exposure time • A well collimated beam • A grid • The smallest possible focal spot • A large focus film distance • A small object film distance • A cooperative, thin patient (!) In reality, a number of compromises must be made
Measurement of Resolution (Sharpness)	• The line pair phantom is made up of strips of lead separated by an air gap equal to the width of the preceding lead strip • Starting at low frequencies (perhaps 1 line pair per millimetre, or lp mm^{-1}), the phantom then progressively decreases the width of the lead strip and the following air gap until high frequencies, perhaps as high as 10 or 14 lp mm^{-1}, are reached

(continued on next page)

NOISE REDUCTION *continued*

Measurement of Resolution (Sharpness) *(contd)*	 **Fig. 7.4** Example of one type of line pair phantom.
Resolution	The size of the smallest object or distance between two objects that must exist before the imaging system will record that object or objects as separate entities. It gives no indication of how the system will record objects of larger dimensions • Or whether they will be visible to an observer • Usually measured in line pairs per millimetre (lp mm^{-1}) • Resolution has a limited value in assessing system performance **Note** Definition • A subjective impression of the details that can be seen in the radiograph • Is difficult to quantify • Should not be confused with resolution
Modulation Transfer Function (MTF)	Allows assessment of system performance at different spatial frequencies (i.e. 'object sizes') • It would be expected that the differences in density of the line pair phantom would be recorded in exactly the same way as the original phantom with the sharp edges clearly delineated • Because of transition density within the image, distinct transition edges are formed which produce a density profile when scanned with a microdensitometer • At low frequencies the transfer of the signal through the system is quite good • As the frequencies get higher the contrast begins to drop rapidly and the pairs of lines become impossible to see • Figures can be obtained for the percentage of accuracy of the transfer of the signal through the system • Therefore the modulation, or altering, of the signal through the system is measured and the modulation transfer function (MTF) for the system is obtained **Fig. 7.5** Reading from an image of a perfectly transferred line pair phantom (100% transfer at all frequencies).

(continued on next page)

NOISE REDUCTION *continued*

| **Modulation Transfer Function (MTF)** *(contd)* |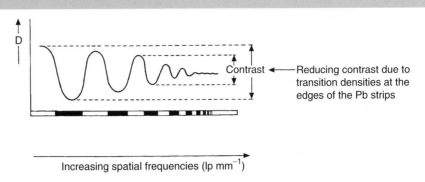
Fig. 7.6 Example of an actual density profile obtained from a line pair phantom showing decreasing information transfer at higher lp mm^{-1}, due to transition densities.

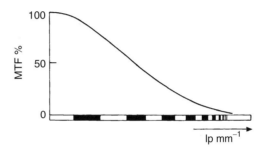

Fig. 7.7 Example of MTF curve, showing loss of information transfer at high spatial frequencies, e.g. at high lp mm^{-1}. |
|---|---|
| **Application** | • Figure 7.8 shows four different films, each with different MTF characteristics
• Film A appears to be most suited to a general radiographic department which requires about 2 lp mm^{-1}
• Film A transfers most information at low and high frequencies
• Film D appears suited to mammography where the demands are greater, and in the order of 4 lp mm^{-1} are required

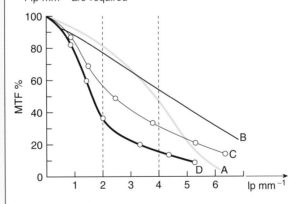

Fig. 7.8 Example of four different MTFs. |

(continued on next page)

NOISE REDUCTION *continued*

Application (*contd*)	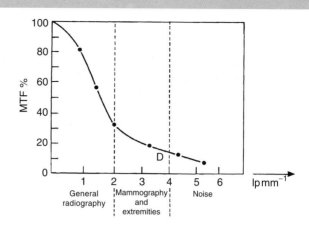 **Fig. 7.9** Suggested limiting resolutions shown on an MTF curve (curve D from Fig. 7.8). **Note** • The minimum size of object which is seen is the signal • Everything smaller than this size is information that is not required and is noise

SHARPENING DIGITAL IMAGE

Edge Enhancement	The use of filters to highlight the boundaries between objects • A filter multiplies all the pixel values by a constant • The values are then added together • The results are then divided by a second figure • The results are then applied to a range of grey scales • Makes the boundaries more conspicuous **Application** • Can aid the identification of small lesions in the body **Note** • Changes the subjective appearance of the image and may result in a loss of information
Frequency Domain Method	• Take the Fourier transform of the image • Multiply the transform by a filter • Invert the filtered transform to get the enhanced image • By increasing the size of the high frequency areas of the image the image becomes sharper

SUBTRACTION TECHNIQUES

To Demonstrate Arterial System	• Digital image of the area of concern is taken
	• The film is digitally reversed so that white becomes black – image A
	• The image is stored
	• A contrast agent is given to the patient
	• An image with contrast agent is taken covering the same area as the first image – image B
	• Image A is digitally superimposed on image B – image C
	• In image C:
	  ○ The background information is cancelled out as black is superimposed on white
	  ○ Leaving the arterial system seen in isolation and therefore more clearly

IMAGE COMPRESSION

JPEG	• Images saved as JPEG files are automatically compressed • This reduces the number of bytes in the image • Reduces the amount of storage space required • JPEG compression uses a lost compression algorithm • Therefore the higher the compression the more information is lost from the image • This can result in a loss of detail or image quality

DEFINITION OF IMAGE STORAGE	
	The ability to store patient information in a format that means that it is secure, can be readily accessed by authorised users only and the information does not degrade over time

STORAGE CRITERIA	

Security	Unauthorised viewing of data should not be possible and therefore:
	
	Passwords
	• Need to be changed on a regular basis
	• Linked to each individual user
	• Use of automated password generators (APG)
	  ○ Hand held device (unique to each person authorised to use the system)
	  ○ Person requests a password
	  ○ APG server sends a password
	  ○ User inputs the password
	  ○ The password is changed every time the user goes onto the system
	
	Firewalls
	• Automatically identify information coming from external sources
	  ○ Either allow information in, e.g., from a GP surgery
	  ○ Or exclude information, e.g. from external viruses
	• Part of the internal network
	• Should be updated at regular intervals
	
	Antivirus software
	• Software packages to protect against
	  ○ Viruses
	  ○ Worms
	  ○ Cookies
	• Viruses, etc. gain access via internet connections including e-mail
	• Software should be updated at regular intervals
	• Regular checks should be run on stand-alone computers with internet access
	
	Individual monitor security
	• Antivirus software should be run at regular intervals
	• Internal security settings should be set at high:
	  ○ Firewall – on
	  ○ Block cookies
	  ○ Block pop-ups
	  ○ Allow automatic updates for firewalls and antivirus software
	• Cookies should be deleted at regular intervals
	
	Removal of external disk drives
	• Consider blocking or removing external disk drives
	• Prevents the introduction of viruses from external computers via CDs and DVDs

Access	Limited to the requirements of each user, e.g.
	• Managers limited to management information
	• Clinicians limited to patient details; all information contained in patient records
	• Receptionists limited to patient's contact details, clinic lists
	• Individual passwords used and changed at regular intervals
	• Automatic record of:
	  ○ Who accessed a file
	  ○ The date and time is was accessed
	  ○ Who added to the file
	  ○ Who deleted part of a file.
	
	Note
	If part of the file is deleted it should remain on the record but show it has been deleted, e.g. with a line through the record

(continued on next page)

STORAGE CRITERIA *continued*	

Access (*contd*)	• It is important that staff:
	  ○ Log off as well as log on to the computer
	  ○ Do not give anyone their password
	  ○ Do not write down their password

Speed of Access	• It is important that patient information can be found quickly and easily • Optical disks allow quick and easy access • But have problems due to the size of radiographic images • Images will be stored on the World Wide Web • On a dedicated site • With a dedicated search engine to recall the information
Stability	• Stored images should not degrade over time • Storage media needs to have a long life and equipment needs to be available to read the image at a later date **Note** New computers cannot read floppy disks, so any information stored on these is no longer accessible • Storing images on the World Wide Web may solve these problems
Backup	• Backup is important in case of breakdown or virus attack • Information should be backed up automatically • A separate copy of all data should ideally be stored away from the main site. If this is not possible, a dedicated room should be used • It should not be stored on the same intranet system
Storage Capacity	• A capacity of 0.6 Gbytes, would be capable of storing all details, reports, film locations, appointments, X-ray room details, registrations, etc. for about 1 million patients • That represents the storage of all patient data (in an average hospital) for about 10 years **But** • 2.5 Gbytes is only capable of storing about 170, 35 × 43 cm chest films • Data compression may be able to reduce storage requirements by as much as 50% • Again storage on the World Wide Web will solve these problems

STORAGE FORMATS

| **Magnetic Tape**
Digital Audio Tape (DAT)
Digital Linear Tape (DLT) | **Construction**
• Plastic tape
• Coated with iron oxide
• The surface can be magnetised
• The tape can be purchased in a variety of widths
• An 8-bit tape will have 9 tracks
  ○ 8 tracks to store data plus 1 track for the computer to check the data

Storage of data
• Utilises the principle that electricity can be on or off
• The information from the computer is in binary (hexadecimal) format
• The signal is made up of a pattern of 'on' and 'off'
• If 'on' hits the tape it becomes magnetised forming a 'spot'
• If 'off' hits the tape it is not magnetised
• The information is therefore built up across the tape
• A frame is a complete data set
• An inter-record gap (IRG) separates each frame

Reading
• Tapehead scans the tape
• Detects the magnetised areas on the tape
• Translates them into a signal to send to the computer |

(continued on next page)

STORAGE FORMATS *continued*

Magnetic Tape *(contd)*	**Advantages** • Used for backing up data • Inexpensive • Large memory, e.g. 5 Gbytes **Disadvantages** • Time taken to access data as patient information may be in different areas on the tape • Tapes have to be periodically rewound to prevent degrading of the magnetic information

Memory Sticks	**Type**
	• A solid state storage device
	
	Construction
	• A chip with a grid of columns and rows
	• Two transistors at each cell (where each area of the grid intersects)
	  ◦ Floating gate transistor
	  ◦ Control gate transistor
	  ◦ Separated by thin layer of oxide
	
	Storage of data
	• Utilises the principle that electricity can be on or off
	• The information from the computer is in binary (hexadecimal) format
	• The signal is made up of a pattern of 'on' and 'off'
	• Initially all cells have a value of 1
	• If an electrical charge is put on the floating gate:
	  ◦ The float gate transistor acts as an electron gun
	  ◦ The electrons from the transistor pass through the oxide layer giving it a negative charge
	  ◦ A cell sensor monitors the charge on the oxide layer
	  ◦ If the charge drops below 50% the cell value changes to 0
	  ◦ The information is therefore built up across the cells
	
	Reading
	• The card is electronically scanned to reconstruct the data
	
	Advantages
	• Small in size
	• Allows fast access to data
	• Easily transportable
	• Plugs into any USB port
	
	Disadvantages
	• Expensive
	• If used on infected machines can introduce viruses, etc. into the hospital system

Optical Disks	

Compact Disk (CD)	**Types**
	• CD-R Compact disk recordable
	• CD-RW Compact disk re-writeable
	
	Construction CD-R
	• Outer protective coating
	  ◦ Lacquer
	• Reflective layer – thin metal
	  ◦ Gold, silver alloy, or silver
	• Recording layer – organic dye
	  ◦ Phthalocyanine or azo
	• Plastic substrate – contains a spiral groove extending from the centre of the disk to the outside edge
	  ◦ Polycarbonate

(continued on next page)

STORAGE FORMATS *continued*

Compact Disk (CD) (contd)	

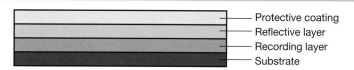

- Protective coating
- Reflective layer
- Recording layer
- Substrate

Fig. 8.1 CD construction.

Construction CD-RW
- Outer protective coating
  - Lacquer
- Reflective layer – thin metal
  - Aluminium
- Dielectric layer
  - Zinc sulphide, silicon dioxide
- Recording layer – phase change alloy
  - Indium, silver, tellurium and antimony
- Dielectric layer
  - Zinc sulphide, silicon dioxide
- Plastic substrate – contains a 0.5 μm (micron) spiral groove extending from the centre of the disk to the outside edge
  - Polycarbonate

Storage of data
- Information written on the disk by 405 nm (nanometre) laser
- The signal is made up of a pattern of 'on' and 'off'
- If 'on' hits the disk the dye layer is heated and darkens
- If 'off' hits the disk the dye remains unchanged
- The information is therefore built up across the disk

Reading
- A 405 nm laser scans the disk from the inside outwards
- Detects the blackened areas on the disk
- Translates them into a signal to send to the computer

Note
A variable motor is used as:
- The diameter of the grove is smaller in the centre than the outer edge
- It ensures that the information is read at a constant rate across the disk
- Speed of reading/writing is dependent on the drive speed of the computer drive

Advantages
- The laser is focused below the disk surface therefore scratches and blemishes are not read
- Any image can be found in about a quarter of a second
- Inexpensive

Disadvantages
- Have a storage capacity of only 650–800 Mbytes
- Are being replaced by DVDs

Digital Versatile Disk (DVD)

Types
- DVD–R
- DVD+R
- DVD–RW
- DVD+RW
- Either single (a recording side and a dummy side)
- Or double-sided (two recording sides)

Construction (single-sided) DVD–R
- Outer protective coating
  - Lacquer

(continued on next page)

STORAGE FORMATS *continued*

Digital Versatile Disk (DVD) *(contd)*	<ul><li>Reflective layer – thin metal<ul><li>Silver, silver alloy, gold</li></ul></li><li>Recording layer – organic dye, e.g. Azo, cyanide, dipyrromethene</li><li>Plastic substrate – contains a 0.5 μm, spiral groove extending from the centre of the disk to the outside edge<ul><li>Polycarbonate</li><li>Number of indentations (pits and lands) between the grooves</li></ul></li><li>Adhesive bond</li><li>Dummy layer<ul><li>Polycarbonate plastic</li></ul></li></ul>**Construction (double sided) DVD+R**<ul><li>Outer protective coating<ul><li>lacquer</li></ul></li><li>Reflective layer – thin metal<ul><li>Silver, silver alloy, gold</li></ul></li><li>Recording layer – organic dye, e.g. Azo, cyanide, dipyrromethene</li><li>Plastic substrate – contains a 0.5 μm, spiral groove extending from the centre of the disk to the outside edge<ul><li>Polycarbonate</li></ul></li><li>Adhesive bond</li><li>Plastic substrate – contains a 0.5 μm, spiral groove extending from the centre of the disk to the outside edge<ul><li>Polycarbonate</li></ul></li><li>Recording layer – organic dye, e.g. Azo, cyanide, dipyrromethene</li><li>Reflective layer – thin metal<ul><li>Silver, silver alloy, gold</li></ul></li><li>Outer protective coating<ul><li>Lacquer</li></ul></li></ul>**Construction of a (single-sided) DVD–RW**<ul><li>Outer protective coating<ul><li>Lacquer</li></ul></li><li>Reflective layer – thin metal<ul><li>Silver, silver alloy, aluminium</li></ul></li><li>Dielectric layer<ul><li>Zinc sulphide and silicon dioxide</li></ul></li><li>Recording layer – phase changed alloy, e.g.<ul><li>Indium, silver, tellurium and antimony or germanium</li></ul></li><li>Dielectric layer<ul><li>Zinc sulphide and silicon dioxide</li></ul></li><li>Plastic substrate – contains a 0.5 μm, spiral groove extending from the centre of the disk to the outside edge<ul><li>Polycarbonate</li><li>Number of indentations (pits and lands) between the grooves</li></ul></li><li>Adhesive bond</li><li>Dummy layer<ul><li>Polycarbonate plastic</li></ul></li></ul>

(continued on next page)

STORAGE FORMATS *continued*

Digital Versatile Disk (DVD) (*contd*)

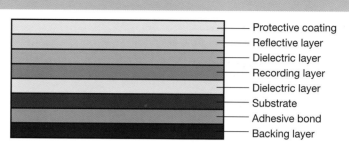

- Protective coating
- Reflective layer
- Dielectric layer
- Recording layer
- Dielectric layer
- Substrate
- Adhesive bond
- Backing layer

Fig. 8.2 DVD–RW construction.

Storage of data
- Information written on the disk by 405 nm (nanometre) laser
- The signal is made up of a pattern of 'on' and 'off'
- If 'on' hits the disk the dye layer is heated and darkens
- If 'off' hits the disk the dye remains unchanged
- The information is therefore built up across the disk

Reading
- A 405 nm laser scans the disk from the inside outwards
- Detects the blackened areas on the disk
- Translates them into a signal to send to the computer

Advantages
- The laser is focused below the disk surface therefore scratches and blemishes are not read
- Have a storage capacity of up to 60 Gbytes and up to 240 Gbytes is predicted
- Any image can be found in about a quarter of a second

Disadvantages
- DVD+ disks will only work on DVD+ equipment
- DVD– disks will only work on DVD– equipment

Magneto-optical Disks

Construction
- A ferromagnetic material with a plastic coating
- With an electromagnet positioned behind the disk

Storage of data
- The disk is scanned twice by a pulsed laser
  - The first scan erases the disk
    - The light varies in intensity and heats up the surface to the Curie temperature
    - Curie temperature is the temperature at which the surface loses its magnetism
  - The second scan enables the electromagnet to 'write' on the disk
- The heating allows the electromagnet to change the polarisation of the disk material

Reading
- A 405 nm laser scans the disk from the inside outwards
- Detects the magnetised areas on the disk
- The reflected light therefore varies in intensity forming the image

Advantages
- 2.8 Mbytes of data can be stored
- Very reliable, as data is automatically checked at the end of writing

Disadvantages
- Writing the data is slow due to the double laser scan

Juke Boxes

Construction
- An electromechanical device

Storage of data
- Contains a number of optical computer disks

(continued on next page)

STORAGE FORMATS *continued*	
Juke Boxes (*contd*)	**Reading** • Enables automatic retrieval of archived material **Advantages** • Allows access to a number of optical disks • Additional juke boxes can be added to the system • Cost-effective **Disadvantages** • Long retrieval time

World Wide Web	**Construction**
	• Potential for a global area network for NHS Data
	
	Storage of data
	• On the network therefore with unlimited capacity
	
	Reading
	• Using a search engine (similar to Google)
	• Search for:
	  ○ Hospital
	  ○ Patient
	  ○ Conditions, etc.
	
	Advantages
	• All patient data available worldwide
	• Images taken in one country would be available in another
	• Unlimited storage
	• Fast access to information
	• Enable researchers to have access to anonymised information
	
	Disadvantages
	• Potential harm from computer virus attack
	• Potential confidentiality problems with computer hackers

TERMINOLOGY	
Asynchronous Transfer Mode (ATM)	A fast and expensive method of setting up a computer network; tends to be used to provide the backbone to a system
Backbone	A physical connection between hubs that carries all data back to the server
Bandwidth	The amount of information in bits per second (bps), kilobits per second (kbps), or megabits per second (Mbps) that can be sent via a communication channel or a network connection in a set period of time, i.e. the speed of the system
Bus	• A set of wires between computers where two signals can travel side by side • The signals can start and finish at any point in the system • The bus has no control of what is sent and when it is sent
Collision	When two or more computers try to send data at the same time down the same network
Deterministic	The method of calculating how long it will take data to travel round a network and how quickly the system can be accessed
Ethernet	A method of setting up a computer network developed by Xerox, using cabling to connect the parts of the system together
Global Area Network (GAN)	Worldwide connecting systems, e.g. • Internet • Telecommunications
Hub	• Equipment that receives information from a network interface card • Re-times the information • Sends the information to its destination
IP Address	• Each node on a system is given its own unique number • Formed by four larger numbers separated by dots, e.g. ◦ 12.345.678.9 • Allows data to be sent to the correct destination
ISDN Connection	A digital telephone line allowing computer connections
Local Area Network (LAN)	A method of linking computers, printers, etc. within a building to enable the sharing of data between computers
Metropolitan Area Network (MAN)	Linking of local area networks over a local district
Modem	Device connecting computers to the telephone system Consists of: • Modulator – converts computer signal to an audio signal • Demodulator – converts incoming audio signal to a digital signal
Network	A method of linking computers, printers, etc. to enable the sharing of data between them

Network Interface Cards (NICs)	• Cards that control the flow of data between a computer and the hub
	• Have collision detection circuits
	• Therefore if two sets of data are sent at identical times from two different machines
	  ◦ One card will automatically delay transmission
	  ◦ Therefore prevent a collision

(continued on next page)

TERMINOLOGY *continued*	
Node	Equipment that communicates in a network, e.g. • Workstation • Printer • Ultrasound equipment

Router	• Equipment that connects:
	  ○ Workstations
	  ○ Networks
	• Increases the capacity of the network

Segment	Section of a network where several nodes are linked together
Server	A method of enabling computers to communicate with each other either by using another computer or software on a computer
Switches	Send information directly to any linked computer in a segment without using the hub
Token Ring	A method developed by IBM, of setting up a computer network using cabling that is joined in a ring
Wide Area Network (WAN)	A method of linking computers to external users via a modem
Wireless System	Used in place of a modem where direct connections are expensive or difficult Uses: • Radio transmitters • Microwaves • Lasers

BASIC LOCAL AREA NETWORK (SIMPLIFIED)	
Equipment to be Linked (Nodes)	• Server (Main computer) • Computers • Workstations • Imaging systems • Printers • Scanners • Modems
Preparation	• All nodes to be networked are identified • Each piece of node is given a unique, identifying, address • Each piece of equipment has a Network Interface Card

Connections	• The equipment is connected to the network via:
	  ○ The network interface card
	  ○ The hub
	  ○ The backbone
	• Using a networking standard
	  ○ Ethernet
	  ○ Token Ring
	  ○ Asynchronous transfer mode

Data Journey	*Example*
	• Information is sent from a computer
	• The network interface card
	  ○ Checks if there is information being transmitted on the system
	  ○ Either transmits data or holds the data back until there is space on the system

(continued on next page)

BASIC LOCAL AREA NETWORK (SIMPLIFIED) *continued*	

Data Journey (*contd*)	• The hub
	  ○ Receives the data
	  ○ Either transmits data or holds the data back until there is space on the system
	  ○ Transmits the data to the backbone
	• The backbone
	  ○ Links together several hubs
	  ○ Either transmits data or holds the data back until there is space on the system
	  ○ Transmits the data to the server
	• The server
	  ○ Stores the information
	  ○ Sends information to routers if required
	• The router
	  ○ Connects local area networks
	  ○ Transmits information between the networks

NETWORK STANDARDS

Ethernet	• Developed by Xerox
	• Linkage is via a bus
	  ○ Connections between computers where two signals can travel side by side
	  ○ The signals can start and finish at any point in the system
	  ○ The bus has no control of what is sent and when it is sent
	• Depends on network interface cards controlling the flow of data
	• Only one single set of data can access the system at a time
	• Although several sets of data can be in the system at any time
	• Simple to install
	• Relatively inexpensive system
	• Not possible to calculate the time taken to send data
	
	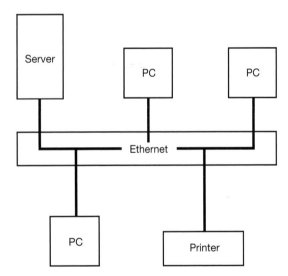
	Fig. 9.1 Ethernet connection.
	
	Developments
	
	10Base5
	• Original system
	• Using thick cable
	• Maximum length 500 m
	
	10Base2 (Cheapernet or Thinnet)
	• Thin coaxial cable used
	• Maximum length 185 m

(continued on next page)

NETWORK STANDARDS *continued*

Ethernet (*contd*)	*10BaseT*
	• Unshielded twisted pair cables
	• Maximum length 100 m
	• Each computer connected directly to the hub
	
	System speed
	• 10 Mbits per second
	  ○ Used for e-mails
	  ○ Access to hospital databases
	  ○ Sending reports
	• 100 Mbits per second – for fast Ethernet system
	  ○ Used for sending images
	
	Note
	• Both standard and fast systems can be used on the same system
	• The system is advancing; speeds of 100 Gigabits per second are now possible

Token Ring	• Developed by IBM
	• Network is joined via a ring of cables
	• Token
	  ○ Small package of data circulates round the system
	  ○ If a computer wishes to send data
	  – The token goes to the computer
	  – Allows full access to the system
	• Data can only be sent if the computer concerned has the token
	• The system is expensive to install
	• The system is described as being deterministic
	• Speeds
	  ○ 16 Mbits per second
	
	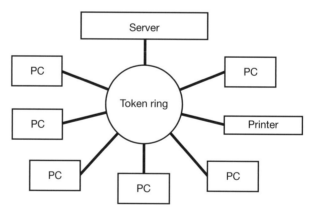
	
	Fig. 9.2 Token ring connections.

Asynchronous Transfer Mode (ATM)	• Expensive to install
	• Used for the backbones of Ethernet systems
	• Transmits data in packets of fixed length 53 byte cells
	• Allows fast switching times due to the small packet size
	• Speeds
	  ○ 155 Mbits per second internally
	  ○ 5 Gbits per second between sites

(continued on next page)

NETWORK STANDARDS *continued*

Asynchronous Transfer Mode (ATM) *(contd)*

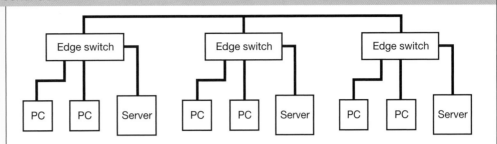

Fig. 9.3 ATM backbone.

DEFINITION OF PACS	
	PACS is a method of storing images in a digital format. Once stored they can be sent to different parts of the hospital and to the wider medical community. Many manufacturers produce systems to enable the transfer of information and the systems they produce contain some or all of the following:

TERMINOLOGY	
Image Identification	• Either a barcode reader or a touch screen for patient identification • Either a barcode reader or a touch screen for cassette identification This can either be: • Downloaded from the central hospital computer or appropriate imaging modality • Keyed in using the computer keyboard *or* • Directly read from a bar code.
Reporting Consoles (Reporting consoles allow instant access to diagnostic images, allowing the decision to be taken immediately as to whether or not additional projections will be required before the patient leaves the department. In addition, current and archived images and previous reports can be displayed alongside each other to give a full clinical picture of the patient's condition prior to reporting)	It is possible to change the image presentation on the monitor with regard to: • *Viewing* several images together • *Viewing* an animated sequence of images • *Tonal conversion* which is the selection of the appropriate contrast and density for the anatomical region under investigation • *Spatial frequency modification* which allows the selective manipulation of an image to eliminate 'blurring' or contrast disparity • *Edge enhancement* as the name suggests, more clearly defines the outline of various bones or organs • *Magnification* allows different parts of the image to be magnified although some systems do not allow the magnified image to be recorded on film • *Measurement, rotation and image reversal* are all possible and in some instances, the operator is able to manipulate the image to produce three dimensional images providing the appropriate software and images are present • *Sound reporting* is the means of dictating and then saving an oral report by using a telephone headset. The recording can then be digitised and stored with the appropriate image. The recording can then be archived, transmitted or replayed at a later date
Remote Consoles	• Viewing stations to retrieve images from the intranet for internal staff • Viewing stations to retrieve information from the internet for external staff • The consoles can be sited throughout the hospital in intensive care units, theatres, accident and emergency departments, teaching units, etc. • The images can be displayed alongside the reports and additional information, e.g. exposure factors, can also be displayed • The use of these consoles can save time as the manual retrieving, transporting and copying of films is no longer required

Central Storage	• A Web server with a database to store the image
	  ○ With automatic deletion after the patient leaves hospital
	• A Web browser
	  ○ For the selection of information by patient name
	  ○ For the selection of images of a specific patient
	• Storage in a DICOM format
	  ○ Allows universal connections to imagers, workstations and external users
	  ○ Using either RAID (Redundant Array of Independent Disks) or CD-R or Digital Linear Tape (DLT)
	• Computerised archiving

Patient Journey	• It is possible to create a database for a patient entering the hospital
	• On this database can then be recorded patient information:
	  ○ Current history
	  ○ Referral letters (which may be received directly from the General Practitioner via an electronic mailing system)
	  ○ Test results
	  ○ Reports
	  ○ An accounting system (to enable rapid and accurate invoicing)

(continued on next page)

TERMINOLOGY *continued*	

Patient Journey (*contd*)	• In addition, it is possible to have the automatic creation of statistical information
	  ○ For stock control
	  ○ Equipment ordering
	The patient information can remain in the system until the patient is discharged from the hospital and can then be automatically stored in the central archive
	• It is possible to store in the order of 2500 diagnostic images on a 5¼ inch optical disk –
	• Or up to 15 000 images on a 12 inch optical disk –
	• Or images can be stored on the World Wide Web, thus saving on storage space

Information Retrieval	Can be based on: • Patient surname/forenames • Date of birth • Imaging number • Condition • Date of imaging production • Or audit value
Hard Copy Images	By networking the system to a laser printer, it is possible to select and then produce hard copies of images and reports for storage in the patient's notes in the conventional way
Modem Links (A modem is the term used for an interface which links units via the telephone system)	It is possible to send images to other hospitals in this country or abroad *Examples* • A patient has had an accident on the continent and then has returned to this country, the images and reports could be transmitted directly to the receiving hospital • If a patient had a condition diagnosed in one hospital and required transferring to a specialist unit; again the images could be sent directly • Some installations allow direct connection to a service engineer to allow the engineer to do quality control checks or to trace and, in some instances, rectify software faults • If faults occur in the hardware, remote fault diagnosis may also be possible, enabling the engineer to order the appropriate components and coordinate the arrival of the parts and the engineer to minimise departmental down-time
Image Security	• Via passwords and defined user groups • External sources receive encoded data
Automatic Updating	Enables the system to automatically access new innovations and technology

THREE DIMENSIONAL IMAGING

	With the advent of workstation systems with their associated increase in power and memory, at an affordable price, software packages have been developed which enable the production of three dimensional images which can be displayed, manipulated and thus allow measurements to take place. In a networked system, it is now possible to manipulate images at stand-alone workstations by, if necessary, downloading power to prevent system overload. Software can be used to manipulate images from ultrasound, CT, MRI, etc. to aid with, e.g. radiotherapy planning, joint replacement surgery, cosmetic surgery and tracing major vessels prior to operations. It is also possible to combine images from several modalities and, e.g. enhance the image or change its orientation

APPLICATION

Volume Measurements	• These can be in the form of quantitative analysis of a defined area, e.g. a tumour • Statistical analysis could be performed • The results can be presented graphically if required
Curved Sections	• By selecting a standard plane through the body which could be transverse, coronal or sagittal, a curved line could be drawn • This could, e.g. follow a blood vessel, and therefore its relationship with the associated structures could be identified

(continued on next page)

APPLICATION *continued*	
Volume Rendered Images	By adjusting the threshold values of an image, either the soft tissue, bone structure or internal organs can be displayed from the same original image
Image Enhancement	This could be used to manipulate an under-exposed image to make it diagnostically acceptable. There is therefore the potential for reducing the initial patient dosage, and by reading, and then manipulating the image from an imaging plate, producing a diagnostic image
Image Analysis	It is now possible to undertake computer analysis of X-ray film images. Some examples of how this technology is being utilised are:
Pronosco X-posure System™ (This is a method of assessing bone mineral density)	• The hand, wrist and forearm are radiographed • The radiograph is digitised using a scanner system • The radius, ulna and three middle metacarpal bones are automatically analysed for porosity and striation • A printout of the bone mineral density estimate is produced
ImageChecker™ (To aid with the screening of routine mammograms)	• The mammograms are taken • The films are placed in an image checker processor which contains a barcode reader, a laser film digitiser and a computer to process the images • The image is digitised • The image is automatically analysed to show regions of interest • Cluster white areas are marked • Dense areas with radiating lines are marked • The original films are reported on in the normal way • The display unit is then activated and the marked images are displayed • The radiologist then reviews the original films in the light of the additional information

DEFINITION OF QUALITY ASSURANCE

	A method of testing digital imaging systems to ensure consistency of results within the computer network. (See also Appendix F: Quality Assurance and Tests.)
Equipment Required	• 1 mm copper filter • 1 straight edge metal strip • Leeds Tor 18 test tool • Leeds test object N3 • Leeds test object GS2 • Leeds test object TO10

TEST FOR LOW CONTRAST SENSITIVITY AND RESOLUTION

Equipment Required	• Leeds Tor 18 test object • 1 mm copper filter • 24 × 30 cm cassette • X-ray tube
Equipment Tested	• Viewing stations • Laser printers
Testing Frequency	Weekly
Testing Method	• Test tool is placed in the centre of the cassette • X-ray tube centred to the cassette • Collimators are fully opened • Copper filter placed next to the tube • Expose plate using: ○ 100 cm, 55 kVp, 45 mAs • Process the film

Results	• View the image on the main workstation monitor
	• The monitor should not be adjusted
	• 18 discs around the inside edge of the circular image should be seen
	  ○ This gives the grey scale of contrast
	• The line pairs in the middle of the pattern are counted
	  ○ Note if the lines appear to merge they are not counted
	  ○ This gives the resolution of the system
	• The test is repeated on the other monitors by the same person
	• The test is sent to the laser printers and evaluated by the same person

Evaluation	• Using the table for testing fluoroscopic equipment
	• Acceptable results are:
	  ○ 16 discs seen, 14 line pairs
	  ○ 2.24 spatial frequency cycles per millimetre
	  ○ A difference of 3 or more discs or 3 or more line pairs indicates a problem, but note that a difference of one could be due to the eyesight of the person doing the test
	  ○ If only one monitor shows a different result the problem is with that monitor
	  ○ If all show a different result the cause could be:
	    – The processor
	    – The cassette
	    – The X-ray tube

(continued on next page)

PHOSPHOR SCREEN CHECK

Equipment Required	• X-ray tube • Cassettes
Equipment Tested	5 random cassettes of different sizes and resolution
Testing Frequency	Weekly
Testing Method	• Cassettes are exposed • Collimators fully opened • Expose plate using: ○ 100 cm, 55 kVp and 6.3 mAs
Results	• Process as usual • View on main workstation monitor

Evaluation	• Look for:
	  ○ Scratches
	  ○ Dirt
	  ○ Artefacts
	• If any damage is seen the cassette should be replaced

LASER BEAM FUNCTION IN THE PROCESSOR

Equipment Required	• A straight edged metal strip • 35 × 43 cm cassette
Equipment Tested	Processor laser beam: • Focus • Movement • Scan line alignment
Testing Frequency	• Every 3 months • After every service
Testing Method	• A straight edged metal strip is placed diagonally over the cassette • Expose plate using: ○ 100 cm, 55 kVp and 6.3 mAs
Results	• Process as usual • View on main workstation monitor • View on one other monitor • Print a copy

Evaluation	• The edges of the metal strip should be:
	  ○ Straight
	  ○ Continuous
	• Wavy edges or gaps indicate
	  ○ Timing problems
	  ○ Laser beam modulation problems

RECEPTOR REPRODUCIBILITY, UNIFORM DENSITY, ARTEFACT ANALYSIS

Equipment Required	2 metal objects to represent artefacts (e.g. paper clips)
Equipment Tested	• Processor • Cassette

(continued on next page)

RECEPTOR REPRODUCIBILITY, UNIFORM DENSITY, ARTEFACT ANALYSIS *continued*	
Testing Frequency	• Every 3 months • After every service
Testing Method	Metal artefacts are placed on two adjacent corners of the cassette • Expose plate using: ○ 180 cm, 55 kVp and 10 mAs
Results	• Process as usual • View on main workstation monitor • The image should be even

Evaluation	• Black or white areas, streaks
	  ○ Repeat the test with the cassette rotated through 180°
	• If the artefact has moved sides
	  ○ Check and clean the cassette
	  ○ Repeat the test
	• If the artefact is on the same side
	  ○ Indicates processor fault
	  ○ Report to service department

SCREEN CLEANING

Equipment Required	Proprietary screen cleaner
Equipment Tested	All cassettes
Frequency	Every 2 weeks
Method	• Only clean screens with the cleaning solution recommended by the manufacturer of the screens • Dust and dirt should be removed with a soft brush, such as a camera lens cleaning brush • For ingrained dirt, use a lint-free cloth and screen cleaner, rubbing in a circular motion without undue pressure • Once the screens have been cleaned, leave the cassettes partially open so the screens can dry naturally **Note** Most screen cleaners contain an antistatic element as static will attract dirt and dust

SOURCE

	Danson D 2002 Quality assurance for computed radiography. Synergy, April

MAMMOGRAPHY IMAGING

Requirements	Images require a wide exposure latitude and sharp definition
Imaging Plate	**Structure** • Differs from a conventional imaging plate by having a transparent support layer • Capable of 50 μm resolution imaging • 10 pixels/mm at standard pixel density and 20 pixels/mm at high pixel density • 18 × 24 cm and 24 × 30 cm format **Fig. 12.1** Mammography imaging plate.
Image Acquisition	**Structure** • Specialist imaging plate • Laser scanner • Reflecting mirror • 2 light guides • 2 photosensors • Enables fast display time **Fig. 12.2** Fujifilm™ dual-side reading system.
Fujifilm Pattern Enhancement Processing (PEM)	**Software** • For mammography • Enables clearer identification of tumours • Enhances microcalcification making it more conspicuous
Kodak Mammography Total Quality Tool (Test Phantom)	**Software** • Analyses reporting software • Predicts common causes of failure • Storage of image test information

DENTAL IMAGING SYSTEMS

Many dental surgeries are still using film and chemical processing but there is a slow change to digital imaging. There are currently two systems available for digital imaging in dental departments

DENTAL SENSORS

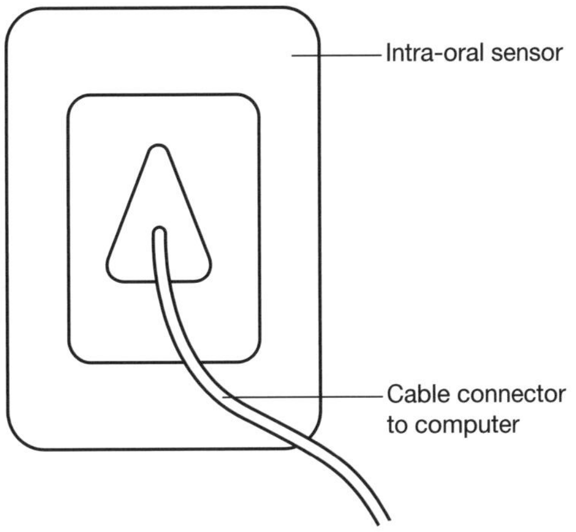

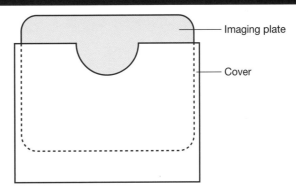

Intra-oral sensor

Cable connector
to computer

Fig. 13.1 Dental – Intra oral sensor.

Structure
- Digital sensor with a waterproof cover
- Disposable cover
- Directly connected to a computer with a cable

When the patient is radiographed
- Image on sensor goes directly to computer screen
- Software available to analyse, manage and store the information
- Can be used for extra oral work

Advantages
- Instant viewing of the image
- Can be integrated into a computerised patient management system
- Image analysis available
- High Image resolution 20+ lp/mm
- No darkroom or chemicals required

Disadvantages
- Sensor is rigid
- Cable may cause problems with positioning
- Careful cleaning required to prevent cross-infection
- Initial cost is high

DENTAL IMAGING PLATES

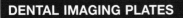

Imaging plate

Cover

Fig. 13.2 Dental imaging plate.

(continued on next page)

DENTAL IMAGING PLATES *continued*

Structure
- Reusable imaging plates
- In light proof pouches
- Disposable cover
- Scanner is directly attached to a computer

Advantages
- Imaging plates are flexible
- Same scanner used for intra oral and extra oral films
- Plates are automatically erased after processing
- Less risk of cross-infection
- Can be integrated into a computerised patient management system
- Image analysis available

Disadvantages
- Plates have a limited life
- Require careful handling to maximise number of times they can be used
- Processing slower than when using a sensor system
- Lower image resolution 14 lp/mm

DEFINITION OF COMPUTED TOMOGRAPHY SCANNING

	Is the process of producing a cross-sectional image of the body by using a collimated beam of radiation that rotates round the patient. Some of the radiation is absorbed and scattered by the body and some is transmitted through the patient and is collected by a number of detectors which are linked to photomultipliers. A signal is then sent to a computer which calculates the amount of radiation absorbed by the patient and reconstructs an image which can then be viewed on a television monitor

TERMINOLOGY

Dynamic CT	When a number of scans are performed in rapid succession, e.g. to demonstrate blood flow
Enhanced CT	The use of a contrast agent to improve the appearance of vessels or organs that are similar in density to the surrounding tissues
Field of View	The part of the scanned plane which may be included in the final image
Helical	Spiral
Image Acquisition	The collection of data in order to produce an image
Image Format	The process of storing an image, on computer disk, magnetic tape, film or on the World Wide Web
Image Manipulation	To digitally change the appearance of the acquired image in order to improve it
Image Reconstruction	The process of generating an image from raw data or a set of unprocessed measurements
Isotropic	Having the same properties in all directions, e.g. density
Matrix	The columns and rows that form a digital image
Mean Window Level	The average range of pixel values in an image
Noise	Anything that distracts from the information required on an image
Nutating Detector Ring	When the detectors vibrate in such a way as to keep the detectors nearest the tube out of the way of the X-ray beam
Pitch	The table movement during one complete rotation of 360° divided by the column width (or slice thickness) **Example** If the table moves 10 mm during one complete rotation and a beam width of 5 mm was used, the pitch value = 2
Pixel	A two dimensional 'picture cell' or 'dot' that makes up the image on a digital display screen
Profile	Line of data
Slice	A section through the patient which is recorded when the X-ray tube and detector make one complete rotation
Slice Interval	The distance between reconstructed slices
Spatial Resolution	The smallest part of an image that can be seen
Translate	Movement in a horizontal direction
Voxel	A three dimensional pixel

(continued on next page)

TERMINOLOGY *continued*	
Window	The range of colour (or grey) scale values displayed on a digital image
Window Width	The range of pixel values displayed in the digital image
HARDWARE	
Gantry	A circular device for holding the detectors
X-ray Tube	A method of producing X-rays which are collimated so that they are aligned to a specific number of detectors
Detectors	• A solid state device containing caesium iodide crystals which collects the amount of radiation transmitted through the patient • Or UFCTM (Ultrafast Ceramic) LSO (Lutetium Oxyorthosilicate) crystal technology
Photomultipliers	• A device for increasing the number of electrons • The photons from the detector hit a cathode which produces electrons which bombard plates and produce more electrons • Used in earlier scanners – replaced by photodiodes
Photodiode	• Simply, a light controlled variable resistance • When dark there is very little current flow • But when the PN junction is exposed to light, current flows in direct proportion to the quantity of light it is exposed to • Solid state devices coated with a fluorescent rare earth phosphor, smaller, more stable and more sensitive and a third of the size of photomultipliers
Housing	• A 'doughnut' shaped structure which contains the X-ray tube and the detectors • With a patient opening (aperture) in the order of 70 cm diameter
Movement	• Originally high tension cables wound round a drum • Disadvantages that the cables had to be 'unwound' after each cycle • Replaced with slip ring and brushes • Gives a constant electrical supply • Therefore allows continual movement during rotations
Table	For the patient to lie on and can move forward at a predetermined distance or at a constant speed to enable the next 'slice' to be taken
Operator Console	Where the operator can determine the settings for the scan
Display Station	For the viewing, analysis, networking and storage of the final image
PRINCIPLES OF IMAGE RECORDING	
Tomographic Principle	• The X-ray tube and detector move together • They rotate round a set point • Structures above and below that point are 'blurred' due to the movement of the tube and detector • The point remains in focus and therefore is sharp

(continued on next page)

PRINCIPLES OF IMAGE RECORDING *continued*

Tomographic Principle (*contd*)	**Fig. 14.1** The tomographic principle.
Tissue Attenuation	As different parts of the body have different densities they absorb radiation to different degrees
Attenuation Coefficient	• Is the measure of the absorption of an X-ray beam along a specific path through a body or substance • Is dependent upon the density and atomic number of the substance • Attenuation coefficient = μ
CT Number	Calculated as: $$\mu \text{ tissue} - \mu \text{ water}/\mu \text{ water} \times 1000 = \text{CT number}$$ • A CT number with a density greater than water is positive • A CT number with a density less than water is negative
Hounsfield Unit (HU)	• A standardised unit for reporting and displaying reconstructed CT values • Water has a nominal value of 0 HU • Air has a value of −1000 HU • Other structures have values relative to water; examples could include Fat −0, Tissue +70, Bone +400, titanium +1000 • A change of 1 HU corresponds to 0.1% of the attenuation coefficient between water and air
Voxel Display	• The voxels in the image are displayed showing the relative density of the subject • Density is determined by the mean attenuation of the tissues in the beam • Scale of −1024 to +3071 Hounsfield units are used • Giving 4096 possible values to be allocated to each voxel
Window	• The range of grey scale values shown in a digital image • Or, the range of colour scale values shown in a digital image
Windowing	• Process of using the Hounsfield units to make an image • 256 shades of grey can be assigned • But the human eye can only determine about 100 shades of grey • The shades of grey can be distributed over a wide or a narrow range of Hounsfield units

(continued on next page)

PRINCIPLES OF IMAGE RECORDING *continued*

Narrow Window	• The grey is distributed over a narrow range of units • The central unit being the average HU for the structure of interest • If the average HU was 50 and a narrow window of 170 was selected then HUs of 85 (half 170) above and below 50 would be used • Therefore the grey scale would extend from −35 to +135 • Any readings below −35 would be pure black • Any readings above +135 would be pure white
Wide Window	• The grey is distributed over a wide range of units • The central unit being the average HU for the structure of interest • If the average HU was 400 and a wide window of 2000 was selected then HUs of 1000 (half 2000) above and below 400 would be used • Therefore the grey scale would extend from −600 to +1400 • Any readings below −600 would be pure black • Any readings above +1400 would be pure white
Scanning	• The process when data is produced by moving the tube and detectors round the patient • Is dependent on the amount of radiation absorbed by the body leaving a quantity of radiation to be detected by the detectors • The operator can set the average HU and the window width so that the signal from the detectors to the voxels (or pixels in earlier units) assigns the appropriate shade of grey to each voxel
Detector Action	• During the rotation of the X-ray tube the detectors record many profiles (or snapshots) • In the order of 1000 profiles per 360° rotation are taken • Each profile is subdivided into sections and fed into 700 individual channels • Each profile is back projected (reconstructed backwards) by computer to show the two dimensional slice through the body that was scanned
Image Reconstruction	*Diagram A* • Taking a snapshot of one point in the scan • The graph shows the total CT numbers per profile as seen by the detectors • A back projection of this data results in a number of lines of different densities **Fig. 14.2** (A) Image reconstruction (simplified).

(continued on next page)

PRINCIPLES OF IMAGE RECORDING *continued*

Image Reconstruction (*contd*)	*Diagram B* • If a second snapshot is taken at 90° to the first • A back projection of this data still results in a number of lines of different densities 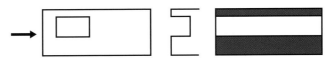 **Fig. 14.2** (B) Scan through 90°. *Diagram C* • If the two images are superimposed • The original image begins to appear If this process is repeated many hundreds of times, a cross-section through the body can be produced. A minimum display would be a matrix of $512 \times 512 = 262\,144$ pixels 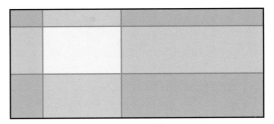 **Fig. 14.2** (C) Superimpose images.
Multiplanar Reformatted Imaging	• A three dimensional image is produced but it is often viewed as a two dimensional image • The advantage is that the imaged can be sliced horizontally or vertically to give a coronal, sagittal or axial view of the patient 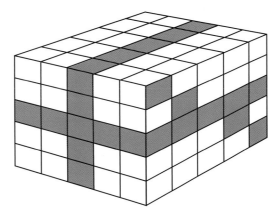 **Fig. 14.3** Multiplanar reformatted image.

DATA MANIPULATION	
Segmentation	• Selection of the tissue of interest • Elimination of data from other organs • Can be done manually or automatically with an appropriate software package
Rendering	• Surface of an organ is assigned a specific shade or colour • Gives the appearance of depth and shade *Surface rendering* • Contours of a specific organ are added together • The surfaces can be highlighted to give an impression of depth • Demonstrates the relationship with adjacent or overlapping structures *Volume rendering* • All the data within an organ or area is assigned a specific shade or colour • Data is manipulated to demonstrate the volume of tissue

DEVELOPMENT	
First Generation Scanner	• A narrow X-ray beam • A single detector • The beam translates slowly across the width of the patient and then stops • The tube and beam were rotated through one degree and the process repeated until an arc of 180° had been completed • Power was supplied to the X-ray tube using high voltage cables wrapped round rotating drums • Reconstruction time was 20 minutes (later 4 minutes) • The image was made up of 'slices' through the body 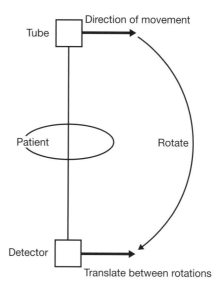 **Fig. 14.4** First generation scanner.
Second Generation Scanner	• A fan shaped X-ray beam • A number of detectors arranged in a row • Each detector collected information for a different angle • The movement was identical to the first generation scanners but through a 30° arc • Reconstruction time 90 seconds • The image is made up of 'slices' through the body

(continued on next page)

DEVELOPMENT *continued*	
Second Generation Scanner (*contd*)	 **Fig. 14.5** Second generation scanner.
Third Generation Scanner	• A wide, fan shaped X-ray beam which extended beyond the edge of the patient • A number of detectors, in two rows, arranged in an arc • The tube and detectors rotated together • The construction was simpler as there was no translational movement • Reconstruction time 10 seconds • The image is made up of 'slices' through the body • Basis for modern scanners **Fig. 14.6** Third generation scanner.
Fourth Generation Scanner	• A wide, fan shaped X-ray beam which extended beyond the edge of the patient • A number of detectors, in two rows, arranged in a complete circle • Only the tube rotates • Originally, the tube was inside the ring of detectors but this resulted in poor geometry and higher patient dose • Solved by using a nutating detector ring

(continued on next page)

DEVELOPMENT *continued*

Fourth Generation Scanner (*contd*)	• Reconstruction time 1 second • The image is made up of 'slices' through the body • More expensive than third generation scanners • More sensitive to artefacts as the relationship between the tube and detectors was not fixed 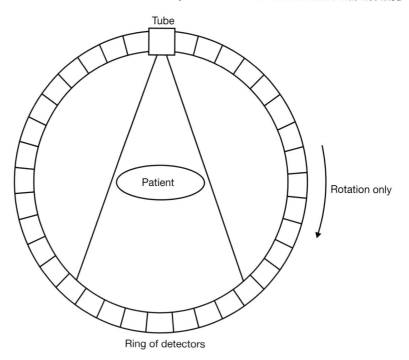 **Fig. 14.7** Fourth generation scanner.
Helical Scanner	• Central ray of the X-ray beam follows a spiral round the patient's body • Collimation of the beam can be varied between 2 mm and 5 mm • The tube and two rows of detectors rotate together at a speed of 60 rotations per minute • Slip rings and brushes maintain constant electrical contact during the scan • The table and patient move slowly and evenly into the gantry until area of interest has been scanned • The pitch can be set between 1.0 mm and 2.0 mm • Reconstruction time is several seconds • Data is collected for the total volume scanned rather than individual slices • It is possible to overlap image construction by manipulating the raw data to reduce artefacts and increase the detection of small lesions

(continued on next page)

DEVELOPMENT *continued*	
Helical Scanner (*contd*)	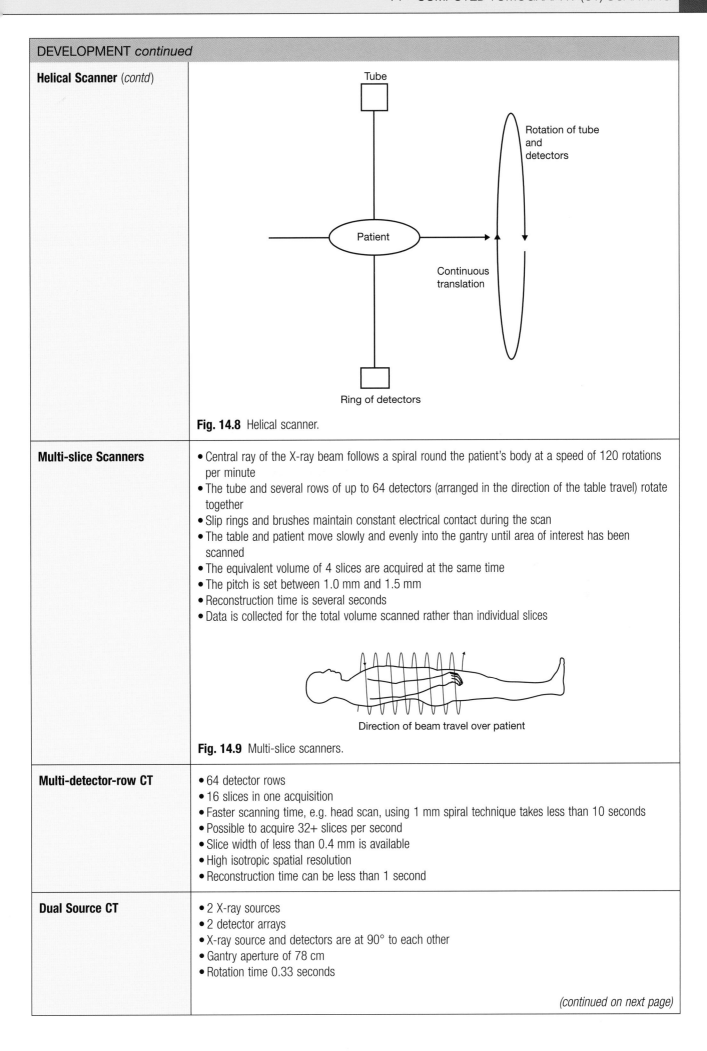 **Fig. 14.8** Helical scanner.
Multi-slice Scanners	• Central ray of the X-ray beam follows a spiral round the patient's body at a speed of 120 rotations per minute • The tube and several rows of up to 64 detectors (arranged in the direction of the table travel) rotate together • Slip rings and brushes maintain constant electrical contact during the scan • The table and patient move slowly and evenly into the gantry until area of interest has been scanned • The equivalent volume of 4 slices are acquired at the same time • The pitch is set between 1.0 mm and 1.5 mm • Reconstruction time is several seconds • Data is collected for the total volume scanned rather than individual slices Direction of beam travel over patient **Fig. 14.9** Multi-slice scanners.
Multi-detector-row CT	• 64 detector rows • 16 slices in one acquisition • Faster scanning time, e.g. head scan, using 1 mm spiral technique takes less than 10 seconds • Possible to acquire 32+ slices per second • Slice width of less than 0.4 mm is available • High isotropic spatial resolution • Reconstruction time can be less than 1 second
Dual Source CT	• 2 X-ray sources • 2 detector arrays • X-ray source and detectors are at 90° to each other • Gantry aperture of 78 cm • Rotation time 0.33 seconds

(continued on next page)

DEVELOPMENT *continued*

Dual Source CT (*contd*)	• Scan range 200 cm • 4 cm volume in one rotation • Acquisition time about 0.1 seconds • Used for cardiac work
Fluoroscopic CT	• Works like a video camera • Allows the acquisition and immediate display of 9 images per second • Images are constantly updated • Uses the same kVp but lower mA than other scanners

SOURCES

Connor S E J, Guest P 1999 Spiral computed tomography pulmonary angiography. Synergy, April

Harvey D 2004 CT evolution. Radiology Today 5(18):August

Hogg P 2005 An overview of PET/CT and its place in today's UK healthcare system. Synergy, December

Patel H, Clarkson L M 2006 MDCT: Practical implementation of a new technology. Synergy, March

Robinson L 1999 Evaluating the colon with CT. Synergy, August

Scally A, Webster M 2001 The evolution of CT technology and its applications. Synergy, March

Smyth J, Hutchinson J 2004 Cardiac CT: A radiographer's perspective. Synergy, October

DEFINITION OF MAGNETIC RESONANCE IMAGING	
	A non-invasive technique that uses radio-frequency radiation in the presence of a powerful magnetic field to produce high-quality images of the body in any plane

TERMINOLOGY	
Acquisitions (Number of Excitations, Signal Averages)	The gathering of enough information to spatially encode one complete data set
Dephasing	When the RF pulse is switched off, the spinning protons go out of phase resulting in a reduction in the received signal
Echo Time (TE)	• Gives the quantity of dephasing that happens between the excitation pulse and the echo • The shorter the echo time, the lower the dephasing, the higher the proton density (T_1) and the better the image
Flip Angle (α)	The degree by which the proton is tipped in relation to the main magnetic field when a RF pulse is applied to it
Fourier Transform	• A method of mathematically changing data, e.g. changing image space to k-space
Gradient Echo	• A basic pulse sequence that only uses magnetic field gradient reversal to re-phase the transverse magnetisation and produce echoes of the magnetic resonance signal • Allows shorter repetition times and faster scanning • Uses flip angles between 0° and 90°
Image Space	An MRI image
Inversion Recovery (IR)	• A basic pulse sequence of 180°, 90° and 180° which inverts the magnetisation and measures the time taken for the nuclei to return to the equilibrium • The rate of recovery depends on the relaxation time T_1
k-space	• The Fourier transform of an MRI image • Gives the frequency and the phase encoding directions
Larmor Equation	At a given field strength, the nuclei of different elements will precess at different frequencies, the equation is used to calculate the frequency of the RF pulse
Larmor Frequency	The rate at which the protons spin when a magnetic field is applied
Magnetic Field Gradient	The loss or increase of magnetic strength over distance controlled by the electrical current passing through the coil • Determines the plane to be imaged • The stronger the gradient the faster the scan or the higher the resolution
Noise	Unwanted electrical signals causing grain on the image
Precession	Is the circular movement of the magnetic axis of a spinning proton which is prescribed when an external magnetic field is applied to the proton

(continued on next page)

TERMINOLOGY *continued*	
Precession (*contd*)	 **Fig. 15.1** Precession.

Pulse Sequence	The bursts of electromagnetic energy produced by the radio-frequency coils
	• Comprises, e.g.
	  ○ Saturated recovery
	  ○ Inversion recovery
	  ○ Spin echo

Radio-frequency (RF) Pulse	A burst of electromagnetic energy at right angles to the magnetic field
Relaxation Time	The time taken for the spinning protons to release the energy obtained and return to their original state
Repetition Time (TR)	The time between the beginning of one radio-frequency pulse sequence to the start of the next, e.g. 300 ms or 500 ms at 1.5 Tesla
Resonance	When an object (a proton) responds to an alternating force (a radio-frequency signal) causing movement
Saturated Recovery (SR)	• When all the longitudinal magnetisation is measured before a 90° radio-frequency pulse is applied • Time consuming procedure • Used for protein density weighted images • Superseded by spin echo sequences
Saturation	The maximum degree of magnetisation that can be achieved in a substance
Signal to Noise Ratio	Image quality = Signal (information required from image)/Noise (unwanted information on an image) Can be improved by: • Increasing the number of signal excitations • Increasing the field of view • Or increasing the strength of the main magnetic field
Spatial Encoding	The prediction of the strength of the magnetic field and the movement of the protons at a set point along a gradient
Spin Echo (SE)	• The reappearance of a magnetic resonance signal after the initial signal has disappeared following a 90° radio-frequency pulse followed by a 180° radio-frequency pulse • Used to detect localised pathology
Spin Polarisation	• The difference between the number of protons that have aligned with the magnetic field and those that have not • Gives the strength of the signal • The more protons that align the stronger the signal

(continued on next page)

TERMINOLOGY *continued*	
T_1 Relaxation Time	• The time taken for the proton spins to release the energy obtained from the initial radio-frequency impulse and return to their natural state • It represents the time required for the longitudinal magnetisation (M_z) to go from 0 to 63% of its final maximum value
T_2 Relaxation Time	• The time required for the transverse magnetisation to reduce to about 37% of its maximum value • Is the characteristic time constant for loss of phase unity amongst spins orientated at an angle to the static main magnetic field
Tesla	• A unit for measuring the strength of a magnetic field • A magnetic flux density of 1 Tesla exists if the force on a 1 metre long straight wire, carrying a current of 1 ampere, is 1 Newton and the wire is placed at right angles to the direction of magnetic flux

HARDWARE

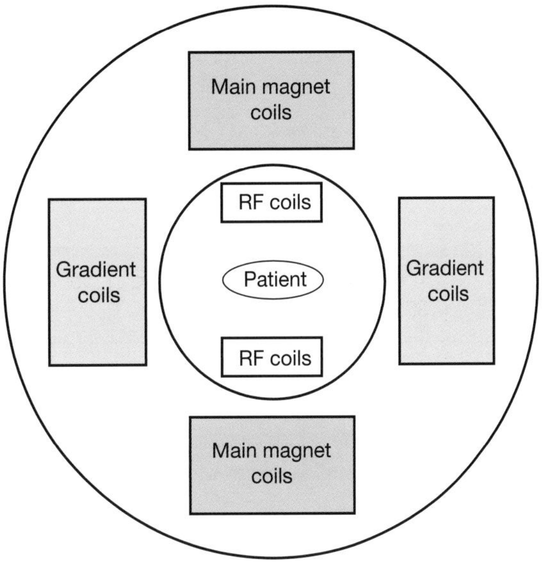

Fig. 15.2 MRI coil position (diagrammatic).

Cryocooler	A closed container: • Condenses the liquid helium vapour • Prevents the need for topping up the liquid helium
Cryostat	A container for: • The coils of the superconducting magnet • A coolant, liquid helium
Gradient Coils (Secondary Magnetic Coils)	Are magnetic coils that are designed to increase or decrease the strength of the main magnetic field • They are usually positioned in three planes • Have a reducing strength along the field, e.g. 1.45 to 1.55 Tesla • The movement of the protons can be predicted • Are used to localise a slice and spatially encode slice information to show the position in the patient and therefore allow focusing on a particular area of the body.
Magnets	Produce the main magnetic field • Low-field strength permanent magnets up to 0.2 Tesla, usually 'C' shaped • Low- to mid-field strength resistive magnets up to 0.35 Tesla (no longer used) • Mid- to high-field strength superconducting magnets 0.5 to 2.0 Tesla, usually cylindrical Magnets have to have strength and straight, parallel lines of force in the iso centre

(continued on next page)

HARDWARE *continued*	
Phased Array Coils	• Receive coils • Produce an even signal covering a large area • Produce high spatial resolution images • Faster scan times ○ Reduce patient movement both voluntary and involuntary
Radio-frequency (RF) Coils	• Produce a fluctuating magnetic field which causes the protons to precess • Detect the RF signal produced by the precessing proton when it turns to align itself with the external magnetic field
Solenoid Technology (ST) Coils	A type of open radio-frequency coil that encloses the area of interest, e.g. a neck coil giving: • Good signal to noise ratio • Better patient comfort • Anatomical coverage in the vertical magnetic field • Larger depth penetration • Imaging extends outside the edge of the coil Vertical magnetic field **Fig. 15.3** Vertical magnetic field.
Surface Coils	Small radio-frequency coils positioned close to the area of interest • Give a better signal to noise ratio • Can only detect a signal at a depth in the patient equal to the radius of the coil
BASIC PRINCIPLES OF IMAGE RECORDING	
Hydrogen	• Has one proton in its nucleus • Is common in the body in the form of water (10^{23} hydrogen protons per ml)

Strong Magnetic Field Applied to the Patient	• Some of the hydrogen protons align to the new magnetic field
	• Field strength used:
	  ○ 0.15 to 1.5 Tesla
	• Earth's magnetic field
	  ○ 5×10^{-6} Tesla
	
	North
	South
	
	Fig. 15.4 Proton alignment when a magnetic field is applied.

Gradient Coils	Determine the plane to be recorded

(continued on next page)

BASIC PRINCIPLES OF IMAGE RECORDING *continued*

Pulses of Radio Waves	• Displace the protons from their new position
	• When the pulse ceases
	  ○ The protons realign
	  ○ They release the energy absorbed as a radio signal of the same frequency

Radio-frequency Coils	• Produce the pulsed radio waves
	• Detects the released energy from the protons
	  ○ Energy is proportional to the number of protons
	  ○ The energy produces a digital signal

Scanning	• To give a 256×256 matrix, 256 phase lines are needed • The slice position is determined by the gradient coils • The lines are determined by the measurement of the relaxation time of the protons following an RF signal
Image	• Signal is analysed by computer • Reconstructed image is displayed as a range of greyscale values

Contrast Agents	*Examples*
	• Water
	• Paramagnetic, e.g. gadolinium compound
	• Superparamagnetic e.g. iron oxide nanoparticles
	
	Advantages of MRI
	• Does not use ionising radiation.
	• Can produce images in any plane
	• Gives good contrast resolution
	• Good for soft tissue imaging, e.g. tumours
	• Can be used for pregnant women but only when essential and without the use of contrast agents
	
	Disadvantages of MRI
	• Due to the magnetic field the presence of:
	  ○ Pacemakers
	  ○ Aneurysms clips
	  ○ Electrical implants
	  ○ Metal implants, e.g. stainless steel
	  ○ Ferromagnetic foreign bodies in the patient
	  ○ Ferromagnetic objects in the room
	Are usually contraindicated due to the potential movement of the object or the heating of the metal by induction, but note that titanium is not affected by the magnetic field
	• Claustrophobia if a closed tube is used
	• Hyperthermia can occur in obese patients due to the radiofrequency energy
	• Noise from the machine can be very high, therefore ear protection is necessary
	  ○ Use of ear protectors
	  ○ The use of noise cancellation systems

DEVELOPMENTS

Cylindrical System with Improved Solenoid Technology (Philips)	• Better signal to noise ratio • Anatomical coverage in the vertical field • Coils form a loop round the body • The anatomy of interest is inside the coil • Sensitivity is in the head to feet direction • 1.0 Tesla open system = 1.5 Tesla cylindrical system • Neck coil 12 cm ST coil does not touch the skin therefore is more comfortable for the patient • 3 × 12 cm ST coil, covers the circle of Willis to the aortic arch

Diffusion Weighted Imaging (DWI)	• Principle
	  ○ In normal tissue the protons in the water move freely
	  ○ Following injury, cells walls absorb water, swell and restrict the movement of the protons
	• An echo plane sequence is followed by two gradient episodes which cancel out plane shift in damaged areas but do not affect the image of normal tissue due to the free movement of the protons
	• The injured areas therefore have a high signal intensity
	• Application
	  ○ Early stroke
	  ○ Early head injury

Functional MRI (Echo Planar Imaging EPI)	• The production of a moving tomographic image
	  ○ Has improved strength and switching of the gradient system
	  ○ Higher resolution with thinner slice thickness
	  ○ Data is collected, processed and stored more quickly
	• The imaging sequence results in:
	  ○ A phase encoded gradient
	  ○ A frequency encoded gradient
	  ○ A phase encoded gradient
	  ○ A reversed frequency encoded gradient
	  ○ The image is recorded during the frequency encoded gradients
	
	Example applications
	• To measure blood flow response when the patient is at rest and during stimulation
	• Investigates the working of the brain
	  ○ Visual, auditory and motor functions
	  ○ Smell, speech, pain
	  ○ Conditions, e.g. epilepsy, neuropsychiatric problems

Magnetic Resonance Angiography	• Using a paramagnetic contrast agent or • Using flow-related enhancement ○ The signal is due to the flow of blood into the imaging plane
MR Guided Therapy	Using MRI to assist with, e.g. • Aspiration cytology • Electrophysiology • Tissue removal using lasers • Cryotherapy
MRI PAT (Parallel Acquisition Techniques)	• Uses array coils (multicoil, phased array receiver coils) • Coils are arranged along the direction of the plane of interest and are used instead of the gradient coils • Less k-space lines are required to form the image with no loss in resolution • If in a 256 × 256 matrix, only half the lines are needed the scan time is halved • Reconstruction uses a coil sensitivity map to reduce artefacts • Therefore produces reduced scan times with no loss of image quality

(continued on next page)

DEVELOPMENTS *continued*

Open Magnetic Resonance Imaging	• Principle
	  ○ No body coil
	  ○ Surface coils are used that transmit and receive
	• Allows scanning in any plane
	• More acceptable to patients, including children and claustrophobic patients
	• Allows guided therapy/intervention procedures
	• In radiotherapy planning, some patients can be scanned in the treatment position

Perfusion MRI	• Measurement of blood flow before, during and after the injection of a contrast agent
	• Can calculate the volume of blood and the time taken for it to pass through an organ
	• Application, e.g.
	  ○ Determine the viability of tissue after an infarct
	  ○ The blood flow associated with and through tumours

Three Dimensional Imaging	• Specialist computer software is used to produce the image • A radio-frequency pulse of a set bandwidth is used to give a slice through the body • Information from an even number of slices is obtained • The data is recorded on a three dimensional matrix • The data can be viewed in any plane **Fig. 15.5** Three dimensional matrix.

SOURCES

Holmes J E, Bydder G M 2005 MR imaging with ultrashort TE (UTE) pulse sequences: basic principles. Synergy, January

Hussain Z, Roberts N, Whitehouse G 1995 The application of T_1 and T_2 and proton density measurements to optimise detection of hepatic metastases using MRI. Radiography Today 61(695):April

Jones T 1998 Gradient echo pulse sequences decoded. Synergy, September

Radiography Technical Support 2006 Solenoid technology improving imaging with open magnets. Synergy, November

Talbot J 2000 MRI artefacts: the good, the bad and the ugly. Synergy, October

Talbot J 2001 What is noise and why is it a problem? Synergy, January

Weal P, Kilkenny J 2003 The practical applications of parallel imaging techniques using standard radio-frequency coils. Synergy, November

Westbrook C 1998 MR advances – the future. Synergy, February

DEFINITION OF NUCLEAR MEDICINE

	The introduction of a specific pharmaceutical (depending on which part of the body is to be targeted), which has been labelled with a radioisotope, into a patient. The gamma rays emitted by the radioisotope are scanned by a detector and the diagnostic image is produced showing the concentrations of the radiopharmaceutical (e.g. a bone scan) or an indication of function (e.g. the glomerular filtration rate of the kidneys)

TERMINOLOGY

Charge Collection	The pooling of electrons across a crystal
Gamma Camera	A large, stationary, scintillation counter, which records the activity over the whole field at the same time. Used to detect pathologies where the physiology of the structure is changed
Gantry	A structure or support, in which the X-ray tube, detectors and associated electronics are housed
Half-life	The amount of time taken for the radioactivity of a radioactive substance to decay by half the initial value. The half-life is a constant for each radioactive isotope
Image Fusion	When a PET (or SPECT) image and a CT image are viewed together by one being superimposed on the other
Pharmaceutical	A drug used in medicine
Photodiode	A semiconductor used to detect light and then generate electricity in proportion to the quantity of light detected
Photomultiplier	Equipment that produces an amplified current when exposed to electromagnetic radiation (light). Photons hitting the cathode produce electrons which in turn hit other surfaces thus producing more electrons, forming a pulse of electricity which forms the subsequent image
Planar	A two dimensional image
Pulse Height Analyser	Receives the signal from the photomultiplier and only produces an electrical signal if the input pulse lies in a predetermined range
Radioisotope	Any isotope that is radioactive. Forms of an element which have the same atomic number but different mass numbers, exhibiting the property of spontaneous nuclear disintegration
Radiopharmaceutical	A drug consisting of a radioactive compound
Scintillation Counter	A number of scintillator crystals in containers, one surface of the crystal is attached to a transparent glass window and the other surfaces are coated with magnesium oxide to reflect light back into the crystal; the back of the crystal is attached to a photomultiplier tube. If a gamma ray hits the crystal, light is produced and some reaches the photocathode of the photomultiplier
Scintillator	A sodium iodide (or caesium iodide) crystal with a thallium activator
Segmented	Divided into sections
Solid State Detector Material	Semi conductor – Cadmium zinc telluride (CdZnTe)
Spatial Resolution	The smallest distance between two objects that can be visually seen on an imaging system

EQUIPMENT	
Pharmaceutical	A drug which is absorbed by a specific (targeted) area of the body
Radioisotope	Technetium 99m ($^{99}Tc^m$) most commonly used • Is a gamma emitter • Has a half-life of 6.02 hours • Is readily available • Is readily combined with pharmaceuticals • Has lower emissions than other types of radiation It is combined with a specific pharmaceutical so that a specific area of the body will take up the radioisotope
Detector – Gamma Camera	Radiation from the patient passes through: **A multichannel collimator** • Parallel lead columns • Absorb extraneous radiation • Only allows gamma rays that are at 90° to the crystal face to reach the crystal **A scintillation counter** • Gamma rays from the patient hit the glass window • Light is produced by the crystal **Photodiodes or photomultipliers** • Detects the light from the crystal • Converts the light to an electrical pulse **Pulse height analyser** • Filters the electrical pulses • Only allows pulses of a predetermined strength to be measured over time • The signal then goes to the computer monitor **Fig. 16.1** The main parts of a gamma camera.
Operator Console	Where the operator can determine the settings for the scan
Display Station	For the viewing, analysis, networking and storage of the final image

DEVELOPMENT

Rectilinear Scanners	• Original scanner • Detector was sodium iodide with a thallium activator connected to a photomultiplier • Detector moved mechanically over the patient • At the same time a light source moved over a film • The whole body can be scanned and the results recorded on a 35.5×43 cm film • Image recorded on X-ray film or paper • Scan time 30 minutes • Motion artefacts a problem (due to breathing) • Superseded by the gamma camera
Gamma Cameras	• The patient is given a radiopharmaceutical and then scanned • The gamma photons from the patient strike a sodium iodide crystal • Photons are converted into light • Passed through photomultiplier tubes • Light changed to electronic signals • Data collection by an analogue camera • Image photographed onto film • Application: two dimensional (planar) imaging and physiology
Mobile Gamma Cameras	• Utilise solid state digital detectors • Silicon photodiodes and segmented caesium iodide scintillators replace photomultipliers • Now possible to scan in near real time • Give two dimensional and three dimensional images
Dual Headed Gamma Cameras (GCPET)	• Utilise solid state digital detectors • Acquire two views simultaneously – 180° apart • Attenuation correction possible • Whole body scan takes 25 minutes • Therefore increased throughput **Advantages** • Cost-effective • Can be used for all gamma camera studies • In addition can be used for PET studies **Disadvantages** • Not accurate in detecting cancerous lesions less than 10 mm
Gamma Probe	Designed for use by a surgeon to detect small quantities of tissue labelled with either Technetium 99m or Indium 111 • Small hand held probe • Tip contains a caesium crystal • Contained in a stainless steel tube • The tube is shielded with tungsten and has clip-on collimators to reduce the radiation to the operator • The tip is angled to make it easier to move • Linked to an automatic analyser • Produces an auditory signal when radiation is detected Application • To detect radioactive tissue • To check if all radioactive tissue has been surgically removed • For lymph node mapping • Localisation of tumours found on PET scans

POSITRON EMISSION TOMOGRAPHY (PET)

Definition	When a positron is emitted it travels a few millimetres then annihilates with a free electron resulting in the emission of two 511 keV photons leaving at nearly 180° to each other. A ring of scintillation detectors are positioned so that they capture the photons and produce a computerised image. Only if two detectors opposite each other register a photon within a nanosecond of each other are the photons registered. They are used in conjunction with CT scanners where the CT scanner shows the anatomy and the PET scanner the function of an organ or tumour, the images being superimposed on each other. Planar or three dimensional images can be produced
Cyclotron	• Used to produce isotopes with a short half-life • A small, self-shielded machine used in a hospital setting **Function** • Uses magnets to accelerate ions towards a target material • To produce a positron-emitting isotope • Which is automatically attached to a pharmaceutical

Detectors	• Several hundred detectors rotate round the patient
	• Detect the simultaneous emissions of the gamma photons
	• Scintillation detectors include:
	  ○ Lutetium oxyorthosilicate (LSO)
	  ○ Bismuth germinate (BG)
	  ○ Gadolinium oxyorthosilicate (GSO)
	  ○ Sodium iodide
	  ○ Ceramic detectors
	• In three dimensional mode there are no metallic collimators between the detectors to allow more gamma rays to be detected

Gantry	• Can be a shared gantry with a CT scanner • The helical CT scan is performed first and then the PET scan • Whole body scan takes 20 minutes

Software	• Image acquisition
	• Processing
	• Reconstruction
	  ○ The CT and PET images can be viewed side by side
	  ○ The images can be viewed separately
	  ○ The anatomical and the functional images are fused together to produce the final image
	  ○ Window width can be adjusted
	  ○ The display colours can be changed
	  ○ Vertical, horizontal and three dimensional sections can be viewed

Radioisotope	*Examples* • Fluorine-18 half-life 110 minutes • Carbon-11 half-life 20.3 minutes • Nitrogen-13 half-life 10 minutes • Oxygen-15 half-life 2 minutes 2 seconds
Radiopharmaceutical	Fluorine-18 fluorodeoxyglucose (^{18}F-FDG)

Application	• Oncology
	  ○ Differentiates between benign and malignant tumours
	  ○ Demonstrates the stage and grade of the tumour
	  ○ Shows the site of the tumour
	  ○ Demonstrates the response to treatment
	  ○ Can demonstrate cancerous lesions below 10 mm
	• Cardiology
	• Neurology

SINGLE PHOTON EMISSION COMPUTERISED TOMOGRAPHY (SPECT)

Definition	A specialist gamma camera which rotates round the patient at 2.8 revolutions per minute and a number of two dimensional images with a slice thickness of 10 mm are taken by measuring the emission of single photons. They can be used in conjunction with CT scanners where the CT scanner shows the anatomy and the SPECT scanner the function of an organ or tumour, the images being superimposed on each other
Gamma Camera	• Collimator contains many thousand parallel, hexagonal channels • Sodium iodide scintillation detectors are used
Gantry	• Contains the gamma camera detector head • Can be a shared gantry with a CT scanner and therefore hold the X-ray tube • Whole body scan takes 15 to 20 minutes

Software	• Image acquisition
	  ○ Approximately every 3 to 6° of rotation
	• Processing
	  ○ Image manipulation possible to remove overlying anatomy
	• Reconstruction
	  ○ Three dimensional images possible
	    – Lower resolution, and increased noise (than planar images)
	    – May be prone to artefacts
	  ○ Resolution 128×128 pixels

Radioisotope	*Examples* • Technetium 99m • Indium 111
Radiopharmaceutical	*Examples* • Tetrofosmin – cardiac work • Hexamethylpropylene amine oxime (HMPAO) – brain scans • Phosphates – bone scans
Application	• Cardiac • Brain • Bone
Limitations	• Incorrect compensation for attenuated photons can cause underestimation of activity • Areas of intense activity can cause streaking and obscure other areas of the body • Can be difficult to locate increased radiotracer activity

SOURCES

Dakin M 2001 Positron emission tomography in the UK. Synergy, November

Griffiths M 2005 SPECT/CT hybrid imaging technology, techniques and clinical experience. Synergy, January

Griffiths M, Aston A, Roberts F 2003 CT 2003 future's bright the future's fusion. Synergy, November

Griffiths M, Holmes K 2002 The development of nuclear medicine equipment. Synergy, November

Higgins R, Smith L, Vinjamuri S 2004 Pancreatic carcinoma and imaging with PET. Synergy, May

Hogg P, Lewington G 2005 An overview of PET/CT and its place in today's UK healthcare system. Synergy, December

Millns M, Owens S, 2001 Unclear nuclear medicine? Not any more! Synergy, February

Moorhouse S 2005 Gamma camera SPET imaging of solitary pulmonary nodes. Synergy, January

Old S E, Dendy P P, Balan K K 2000 Preliminary experience in oncology of positron emission tomography with dual headed gamma camera. Radiography 6:11–17

DEFINITION OF ULTRASONOGRAPHY	
	Ultrasonography is the formation of a visible image from the use of ultrasound. A controlled beam of sound is directed into the relevant part of the body and the reflected ultrasound is used to build up an electronic image of the various structures which can be viewed on a monitor

EQUIPMENT	
Piezoelectric Crystal	• Quartz crystal • When electric current is applied it vibrates and emits sound waves • When a sound wave hits the crystal it emits an electric current
Transducer (Probe)	• Produces and sends sound waves • Receives reflected echoes from boundaries between tissues • Has a sound-absorbing backing to stop sound being reflected from the probe • An acoustic lens to focus the sound waves • Shape of the probe gives the field of view (footprint) • Frequency of the sound wave determines the depth the wave will travel and the image resolution • The higher the frequency the better the resolution (but more of the beam is absorbed by the tissues therefore the depth of penetration of the beam is reduced) • High frequencies (7.5 megahertz, MHz) are used for superficial organs, e.g. breast and thyroid • Lower frequencies (3.5 megahertz, MHz) for the abdomen • Can contain one or more than one crystal element • Each crystal has its own electrical circuit • In multiple element probes the individual crystals can receive signals at different times • Smaller probes can be used in the vagina, rectum, oesophagus, etc.
Transducer Pulse Controls	**Allow the setting of:** • The frequency of the pulses • The time of the pulses • The scan mode of the machine
Central Processing Unit	**Contains** • A computer – containing a microprocessor and memory • Amplifiers • Power supplies to the microprocessor and transducer **Function** • Sends electrical currents to the transducer • Receives electrical pulses from the transducer – created by the returning echoes • Processes the data • By using the speed of sound through tissue (1540 metres per second) and the time taken for the echo to return • Displays the image on the monitor • Stores the final image
Display	**Can demonstrate** • Shades of grey • Colour • Movement • Two dimensional images • Three dimensional images • Surface rendering • Transparency mode • Real time images

TERMINOLOGY

Acoustic Impedance	• A value given to a substance • Is calculated by multiplying the density of the medium by the velocity of the ultrasound travelling through the medium • It is independent of frequency • When a sound wave hits a substance with a different acoustic impedance part of the wave is reflected back
Acoustic Window	• An area of the body used to allow imaging of underlying structures, e.g. the spaces between the ribs, the liver
Aliasing	• When high velocities in one direction appear as high velocities in the opposite direction • Occurs when an analogue signal is sampled at a frequency which is lower than half its maximum frequency • All the frequency above half of the sampling frequency is projected below the base line (backfolded) in the low frequency region causing artifacts on the image
Amplitude	• The maximum value of either positive or negative current or voltage that occurs on an alternating current waveform • The magnitude (height) of the ultrasound beam • The ultrasound pulse is very brief so the power values arranged over a period of time will be low compared to peak intensity
Coupling Gel	• A gel put on a patient's skin to exclude any air between the transducer and the skin surface • Done to enable the transmission of ultrasound waves between the transducer and the patient
Doppler Effect	When imaging a moving object: • The frequency of the reflected beam is changed by the movement • If the object is moving towards the probe the frequency will be increased • If the object is moving away from the probe the frequency is decreased • The speed of change of the frequency indicates how fast the object is moving
Doppler Scanner	• Equipment used to monitor a moving substance • Measures the change in frequency of the reflected echoes to determine the speed of movement of the object, e.g. the flow of blood or the beating heart
Echo	• The reflection of an ultrasound wave back to the transducer • Occurs when the beam hits a surface at right angles
Fourier Transform	• A method of mathematically changing data, e.g. changing spatial data to frequency data • Spatial data gives the position of the varying intensities (brightness) across an image • Frequency data is number and frequency of sine and cosine waves forming the image
Frequency	• The number of cycles of alternating current that occur in one second • Measured in Hertz (Hz) • Ultrasound is frequencies beyond 20 kilohertz (kHz)
Nyquist Theorem	• States that an analogue signal waveform may be reconstructed without error from a sample which is equal to, or greater than, twice the highest frequency in the analogue signal, e.g. to digitally convert a 2 MHz signal a sample must be taken at 4 MHz
Phased Array	• A sector field of view with multiple transducer elements • Formed in precise sequence and under electronic control • This gives a wide field of view using a small transducer • Used in, e.g. cardiac or paediatric head scans

(continued on next page)

TERMINOLOGY *continued*	
Piezoelectric Effect	When an electric current is produced by certain materials when pressure is applied to their surface
Pixel	• Value stored in the memory of a digital scan converter • Dictates the shades of grey on the monitor • Picture cell • The dots which can be used by a character on a digital image display screen • The smaller the pixel the greater the image quality
Probe (Transducer)	• A hand-held instrument • Composed of multiple elements of piezoelectric material each with its own electrodes
Pulse Repetition Frequency	The number of pulses occurring in one second expressed in kilohertz (kHz).
Rarefaction	The opposite of compression
Real Time Scan	• The image is updated after each ultrasound sweep • Therefore movement can be seen on the image
Scattering	• If the ultrasound encounters air in the bowel the beam will be scattered in all directions causing artefacts on the image which results in a non-diagnostic scan • If ultrasound encounters rough surfaces or small objects it will also be scattered
Sound Wave	• The result of mechanical energy travelling through matter as a wave • Producing alternating compression and rarefaction resulting in vibration • The rate of vibration is measured in hertz (Hz)
Three Dimensional Ultrasound	• The creation of a computerised, reconstructed image which represents the anatomical structure being investigated, e.g. used to visualise the fetal face and the adult heart valves
Ultrasound	• Sound waves with a frequency of over 20 000 Hz • Not audible to the human ear • Diagnostic ultrasound uses 1–10 MHz frequencies
Voxel	A three dimensional pixel

DEVELOPMENT

'A' Scan	• A one dimensional display • Shown as a graph • The amplitude of the returning echo on the vertical axis • The time of the returning echo on the horizontal axis

'B' Scan	• Good to demonstrate anatomy
	• Poor for vessels
	  ○ Partial volume averaging due to slice thickness
	  ○ Thermal noise
	  ○ Grating lobes
	  ○ Reverberations

Two Dimensional B Scans	• Obtain a rapid series of slices through the body • Slices are displayed in sequence • Gives a real time image composed of pixels • When a new image is stored the value of the pixel in the memory is updated and the image changes (real time scanning) therefore one frame equals one image • In freehand systems the spacing of the planes depends on the speed the probe is moved • If too fast there will be insufficient slices to reconstruct the image

(continued on next page)

DEVELOPMENT *continued*	
Two Dimensional B Scans (*contd*)	• Difficult to assess volume • Assumes objects have regular shapes and the axes are measured • The volume is then calculated mathematically • Two dimensional images can be difficult to interpret
Three Dimensional Scanning	• Aim is to acquire a series of two dimensional slices through a volume of tissue • Each slice is adjacent to the previous slice • The images are stored in the memory as voxels • Each voxel represents the signal from a specific volume of tissue • Therefore a slice can be taken through the volume in any direction • The exact relationship of the two dimensional slices must be maintained to give an accurate three dimensional image **Fig. 17.1** Diagrammatic representation of a three dimensional volume of tissue.
Freehand Three Dimensional Scanning	• The probe with the position-sensing device attached is operated manually • Therefore the transducer must be moved in a smooth and regular manner • Information on space location and orientation is sent to the position sensor **Advantages** • The equipment can be added to an existing system • A normal probe is used • It is possible to scan through a small acoustic window • Information can be obtained by rotating an inserted probe **Disadvantages** • The image planes are not in a constant relationship • Overlapping of the scanned planes may occur • Spacing of the planes depends on the speed the probe moves • If the probe is moved too quickly insufficient slices will be captured to ensure accurate image reconstruction
Mechanical Three Dimensional Scanning	• A specialist probe is used to give precise movement • Two dimensional images are acquired at predetermined intervals • During the acquisition process the probe is manually held in a stationary position and moves in an arc • Or the transducer can move in a linear direction when the scanner head is mechanically driven over the area of interest **Advantages** • No overlap of the scanned planes • The angular relationship between the planes is constant **Disadvantages** • The probe is very large • It has limited use if the acoustic window is small

(continued on next page)

DEVELOPMENT *continued*	
Viewing the Three Dimensional Image	**Two dimensional slices** • Most systems give a two dimensional display • Different perspectives can be viewed horizontally or vertically to give a coronal, sagittal or axial view of the patient **Surface rendering** • Requires distinct boundaries to be recognised by the system, e.g. fluid and tissue • The area being imaged must not move during the acquisition **Transparency mode** • Projections 'inside' structures, e.g. the fetal skeleton • Requires distinct acoustic properties between adjacent structures, e.g. bone and tissue
The Advantages of Three Dimensional Scanning	• Time saving – once stored the image can be manipulated • Different planes can be viewed • Volume analysis can be undertaken – important to show small changes • Teleradiology is possible • It is possible to see special relationships in three dimensions, e.g. in obstetrics showing the fetus to the parents **Application** • Echocardiography • Obstetrics • Urology • Vascular work
Doppler Ultrasound	• Demonstrates movement, e.g. blood flow in vessels • Using the Doppler effect
Continuous Wave Doppler	• Transducer has two crystals • One to send echoes and one to receive echoes • Audible sound • Either on an analogue recorder or • Spectral parts analyser – separates the signal into the various parts and assigns importance to each part • Analysis by fast Fourier transform **Advantages** • High sensitivity to low velocities • Detection of high velocities without aliasing **Disadvantages** • Cannot distinguish between sending and receiving signals and extraneous echoes • Does not produce a precise image
Pulsed Wave Doppler	• Uses a pulsed echo system • The transducer sends and receives the signal • Sends in short bursts • Receives when not sending • Return signal is 'gated' – therefore only information from a predetermined depth is transmitted • The choice of gate is determined by the Nyquist Theorem **Advantages** • Due to gating, unwanted structures are eliminated from the image **Disadvantages** • Cannot exceed one half pulse repetition frequency or aliasing will occur

(continued on next page)

DEVELOPMENT *continued*	
Colour Flow Duplex	• Combines B scanning with Doppler and colour to demonstrate motion, direction and velocity • Superimposes a colour image of moving blood over the real time scan • Colour gives the direction of flow • Intensity gives velocity strength • Linear or phased array transducers • Signal analysed by: ○ Amplitude ○ Phase – describes the direction and presence of motion ○ Frequency shift – velocity of motion shown with various colour intensities ○ Non-moving objects – shown as grey, the shade depends on signal strength
Tissue Harmonic Imaging (THI)	• Sound wave becomes distorted as tissue expands and contracts • At certain energy levels additional frequencies are generated called harmonics • Harmonics can be two or three times the frequency of the original sound wave • Travel from the originating tissue to the transducer **The harmonic signal** • Is weaker than the original sound wave • Purer than the original as it has less noise because: ○ It only travels from the tissue to the transducer ○ Can be isolated by filtering out the original signal • Demonstrates enhanced contrast and grey tone differences **Application** • Scanning structures in the middle distance range
Micro Vascular Imaging (MVI) Software	• Pulse-inversion harmonic ultrasound • Images individual micro-bubbles • Captures and stores 10 images per second • Processing techniques remove noise and subtract background information • Used to identify angiogenesis (growth of a network of blood vessels that indicates a tumour)
SonoElastography Software	• Tumours and some inflammatory conditions can lead to loss of tissue elasticity • This technique demonstrates changes in tissue elasticity • Relative elasticity is automatically calculated and a colour overlay is produced on a conventional B mode scan, e.g. stiffer tissue is blue, more elastic tissue is red or benign tumours green, malignant tumours are blue
Real-time Virtual Sonography (RVS) Software	• A magnetic positioning unit detects the position (spatial location and orientation) of the transducer • Calculates the multiplanar construction images from the stored data • At the beginning of scanning, position adjustment is done at the xiphoid process • Displays on one monitor: ○ Real time ultrasound image ○ Corresponding CT or MR image from a stored data set **Used for:** • Direct comparison of lesions • Monitoring of intervention procedures

SOURCES

Baines P 2000 3D ultrasound; how does it work and what is it used for? Synergy, March
Hughes J 2001 3D ultrasound imaging; an expanding technique. Synergy, October
Powers J 2003 Micro Vascular Imaging (MVI). Synergy, April

INTRODUCTION TO WEB PAGE DESIGN

With the growth of the internet, more and more departments are creating their own websites. This section discusses the information required for readers to create and maintain their own departmental website. The final website should be clear to read and accessible to all, it should be able to be quickly downloaded and easy to navigate round. Remember that the UK's Disability Rights Commission found that if a site is easily accessible to a disabled user then it will be a third quicker for an able-bodied person to complete tasks on the site

PREPARATION

Who is the website for?	• Staff • The public • Patients • Healthcare professionals • Other organisations
Why is it being produced?	• To give information • To raise the profile of the department • To answer questions from interested parties
When will it be maintained?	• Daily • Weekly • Monthly
What will be included?	• Contact details • Departmental information (location, etc.) • Appointment booking/cancellation • Radiation regulations • Referral procedures • Information about specific procedures • Who's who in the department • Comments/complaints procedure • Clinical Governance issues • Academic research • Links to other websites
Illustrations?	• Size • Download time • Confidentiality
Accessibility?	Accessible for the: • Visually impaired • Hard of hearing • Elderly Can be achieved by using Cascading Style Sheets

EQUIPMENT REQUIRED

• Web space • Web host • Web name • Web publishing software • Internet access	Use of Hospital site and host name

BASIC DESIGN

Text
• Use clear and simple language
• Consider using bullet points
• Keep pages short
• Left justify pages (easier to scan)
	A simple test:
	• Ask a 10–12 year old to look at the page:
	  ○ Do they understand it?
	  ○ Do they find it easy to navigate?
	• If not, look at redesigning to make it accessible for all users

Font • Main page – consider using Font size 12 pt • Use scripts that are clear to read	Think about using Arial rather than Vivaldi or Times New Roman
Colour • Do not rely on colour alone to provide information • Try to have good contrast between print and background	• Green links may not be read by the visually impaired or people who are colour blind • Contrast is critical for people who are visually impaired and colour blind. Think about using blue, yellow, white and black • Use text as well, or use shapes or texture
Images • Save images as jpeg files to reduce the memory of the image • Consider compressing images using image editing software	People tend not to use websites that take a long time to download, the larger the file the longer it takes to download and not all users will have Broadband

Disabled Access
Can your website be accessed by using:
• A mouse
• Keyboard
• Voice input
	• Test your completed website by navigating with just the keyboard – can you access all areas?
	• Consider using Cascade Style Sheets as these enable different pages to be presented in different styles:
	  ○ On screen
	  ○ In print
	  ○ By voice
	  ○ Braille-based tactile equipment

CREATING THE SITE

Planning	
The Content of the Home Page Brief introduction and topic menu	Title and introductions are important as the first few words are used by Search Engines to locate your site

(continued on next page)

CREATING THE SITE *continued*

Menu Topics These define the subject areas on the web page	Always have an option to return to the Home Page or Main page
Hyperlinked Pages Give details of the topics covered on the site	Bullet point lists are easier to scan than long, wordy paragraphs
Setting up the Site	
Web Publishing Software • Needed to design the site • Wizards are easy to follow	Do not forget to Password-protect the site to prevent unauthorised access
Points to Note	
• An e-mail address can be included for responses • Use 'Insert-Break' for normal sized line breaks • Your Home Page should be in 'index.htm' • Use 'Format–Shared Borders' to place a list of 'Hyperlinks' in all your pages	• Do you have the time to respond promptly to queries? • Enter/Return produces large line breaks

UPLOADING A SITE

Example of Uploading a Site using Microsoft FrontPage	• MS FrontPage – File – New – More Website templates – Personal Website – OK • Go back into Windows Explorer – My Websites • Rename the new site 'Imaging Site date' • Upload the new site

GENERAL LEGISLATION

	The following are some of the regulations that apply to the UK, and other readers should check the local regulations for their own country. Only an outline of the main contents have been given, as the main texts are readily available on the internet
Human Rights Act 1988	**Areas of note** • Article 2 Right to life • Article 5 Right to liberty and security • Article 8 Right to respect for private and family life • Article 9 Freedom of thought, conscience and religion • Article 10 Freedom of expression • Article 14 Prohibition of discrimination
Data Protection Act 1998	**Eight basic principles:** Personal information must be: 1. Processed fairly and legally 2. Obtained for limited purposes only 3. Adequate, relevant and not excessive 4. Accurate 5. Not kept longer than is necessary 6. Processed according to an individual's rights in the Act 7. Kept secure 8. Not transferred abroad without adequate protection
Freedom of Information Act 2000	**Gives the power to individuals to:** • Ask a public organisation for information on specific subjects **Covers all NHS organisations who have to:** • Have a publication scheme for releasing information • Tell applicants whether or not they hold information not covered under the publication scheme • Disclose information to applicants, providing it is not exempt under the Act
Health and Safety at Work Act 1974	**The Act outlines the general duties that:** • Employers have towards employees and members of the public • Employees have to themselves and to other employees
The Management of Health and Safety at Work Regulations 1999	**Requires employers to:** • Carry out a risk assessment • Make arrangements for implementing the measures identified by the risk assessment • Appoint competent people to help to implement the arrangements • Set up emergency procedures • Provide information and training • Work with other employers sharing the same workplace
Health and Safety (Display Screen Equipment) Regulations 1992	These regulations cover employees who use display screen equipment daily and for continuous spells of 1 hour or more at a time **The key duties of employers are:** • To identify areas where display screen equipment is used • To identify which staff use the equipment and for how long • To assess the risks to users (if any) and reduce the risks where appropriate • To ensure that any new work stations meet the health and safety requirements • To make sure that staff have adequate breaks and changes of activity • To provide users with eye and eyesight tests, if appropriate • To ensure that any users receive adequate training and information concerning safe working practices

THE FOLLOWING ARE CONCERNED WITH RADIATION

Health and Safety (Display Screen Equipment) Regulations 1992 (*contd*)	• The Medicines (Administration of Radioactive Substances) Regulations 1978 • The Radioactive Substances Act 1993 • The Ionising Radiations Regulations 1999 • The Radioactive Material (Road Transport) (Great Britain) Regulations 2002 • The Ionising Radiation (Medical Exposure) Regulations 2000 • Notes for the Guidance on the Clinical Administration of Radiopharmaceuticals and Use of Sealed Radioactive Sources 2006
The Medicines (Administration of Radioactive Substances) Regulations 1978 **The Medicines (Administration of Radioactive Substances) Amendment Regulations 1995**	**Main areas** • Prior authorisation to provide protection for the patients during the clinical use of radioactive substances • Prior authorisation to provide protection for the volunteers during research in the use of radioactive substances • Indirectly, the protection of staff when using radioactive substances • Criteria for the issue and renewal of a certificate to administer radioactive substances • Only a doctor or dentist holding a certificate issued by the Health Minister or people working under the direction of the doctor or dentist can administer radioactive substances • The amendment regulations make some administrative changes to the regulations
The Radioactive Substances Act 1993	**Covers** • Registration of use of radioactive material and mobile radioactive apparatus • Disposal of radioactive waste • Duty to display documents
The Ionising Radiations Regulations 1999	**Main areas** *General principles and procedures* • Authorisation of specific practices • Notification of specified work • Prior risk assessments • Restriction of exposure • Personal protective equipment • Maintenance and examination of engineering controls and personal protective equipment • Dose limitation • Contingency plans *Arrangements for the management of radiation protection* • Radiation protection adviser • Information, instruction and training • Cooperation between employers **Designated areas** • Designation of controlled or supervised areas • Local rules and radiation protection supervisors • Monitoring of designated areas *Classification and monitoring of persons* • Designation of classified persons • Dose assessment and recording • Estimated doses and special entries • Dosimetry for accidents, etc. • Medical surveillance • Investigation and notification of overexposure • Dose limitation for overexposed employees

(continued on next page)

THE FOLLOWING ARE CONCERNED WITH RADIATION *continued*

The Ionising Radiations Regulations 1999 *(contd)*	**Arrangements for the control of radioactive substances, articles and equipment** • Sealed sources and articles containing or embodying radioactive substances • Accounting for radioactive substances • Keeping and moving radioactive substances • Notification of certain occurrences • Duties of manufacturers, etc. of articles for use in work with ionising radiation • Equipment used for medical exposure • Misuse of or interference with sources of ionising radiation *Duties of employees* • Approval of dosimetry services • Defence on contravention • Exemption certificates • Extension outside Great Britain • Modifications relating to the Ministry of Defence
The Radioactive Material (Road Transport) Regulations 2002	**Main areas** • Transport of radioactive material • Radiation protection, safety programmes and information to the public • Activity limits and material restrictions • Transport controls • Further responsibilities of consignors and carriers • Requirements for radioactive materials, packaging and packages • Test procedures • Approval requirements for designs and shipments • Approval certificates • Radiological emergencies and intervention arrangements
The Ionising Radiation (Medical Exposure) Regulations 2000 Amended 2006	**Concerned with** • Storage and disposal of radioactive waste
Notes for the Guidance on the Clinical Administration of Radiopharmaceuticals and Use of Sealed Radioactive Sources 2006	**Main areas** • Criteria for obtaining certificates to administer radiopharmaceuticals and sealed radioactive sources • Diagnosis • Treatments • Research requirements • Investigations in children and young persons • Conception, pregnancy and breast feeding • Thyroid blocking **The Appendices cover:** • Routine procedures, activities and doses • Calculating radiation doses • Sample size and power calculations • Training and experience • Additional Acts and Regulations • Certification process under the MARS Regulations 1978 • Communicating risk to Local Research Approved Bodies and research subjects

LEGISLATIVE REQUIREMENTS FOR DEALING WITH THE USE AND DISPOSAL OF PHOTOGRAPHIC CHEMICALS ARE DEALT WITH UNDER THE FOLLOWING ACTS

	• Control of Substances Hazardous to Health (COSHH) Regulations 1999 • The Personal Protective Equipment (EC Directive) Regulations 1992 • Environmental Protection Act (EPA) 1990 • Water Act 1989 • The Chemicals (Hazard Information and Packaging for Supply) Regulations 1994 (amended 1999) • Pollution Prevention and Control Act 1999 • European Packaging Waste Directive 1994
COSHH Regulations	**Regulation 3** • The employer is responsible (so far as it is reasonably practicable) for all people who may be affected by substances whether or not they are directly employed **Regulation 6** Assessment of health risks created by work involving substances hazardous to health • An assessment of the risks of any substance hazardous to health should be carried out before the employee is asked to work with the substance • The employee can review an assessment if it is thought to be no longer valid **Regulation 7** Prevention or control of exposure to substances hazardous to health • The emphasis is placed on preventing injury happening • Personal protective equipment must be provided • With regard to inhalation of chemicals the occupational exposure standards (OESs) must not be exceeded • Lists of OESs are published by the Health and Safety Executive in leaflet EH40 which is updated annually • Two exposure limits are given for each chemical: the long term (8 hours weighted average) and the short term (10 minutes weighted average) • OESs are basically the vapour pressures over a given time and are measured in parts per million • Regulation 7.5.b. requires the employer to take action and, as soon as is reasonable, remedy the situation if it is identified that the OES has been exceeded To reduce the quantity of fumes • Ensure there is adequate ventilation (in the order of 12–15 air changes per hour) • Duct processors to the outside air • Use of low temperature and 'low fume' chemicals • Good drainage • The proper positioning of silver recovery equipment • The safe and correct handling of chemicals **Regulation 8** Use of control measures • Employers should ensure that substances are used in the correct manner • Employees should ensure that they use the equipment correctly • Report any defects to their employer as soon as possible **Regulation 9** Maintenance, examination and test of control measures • Non-disposable, personal protective equipment should be checked at 'suitable intervals' by examination and, where necessary, tests • A record should be made of the date, the examination/test, the results and, if appropriate, any repairs undertaken • The records should be kept for 5 years from the date they were made **Regulation 10** Monitoring exposure at the workplace • Ensuring that the occupational exposure limits were not breached for those substances present in processing chemicals

(continued on next page)

LEGISLATIVE REQUIREMENTS FOR DEALING WITH THE USE AND DISPOSAL OF PHOTOGRAPHIC CHEMICALS ARE DEALT WITH UNDER THE FOLLOWING ACTS *continued*	
COSHH Regulations (*contd*)	**Regulation 11** Health surveillance • Although modern chemicals have a reduced risk staff should still be monitored **Regulation 12** *Information, instruction and training* The employer must provide: • Instruction and training in the safe use of processing chemicals • Including information about the health hazards • The precautions which should be taken • If an OES is exceeded, the employee (or their representative) should be informed

The Personal Protective Equipment (EC Directive) Regulations 1992	Personal protective equipment is provided which is of an approved standard
	• For the:
	  ○ Manual mixing of chemicals
	  ○ Wiping up of chemical spillages
	  ○ Changing of processing chemicals
	  ○ Cleaning of machines
	• Would include:
	  ○ Protective clothing
	  ○ Gloves
	  ○ Eye protectors
	  ○ The use of automatic chemical mixers should be considered

Environmental Protection Act (1990)	**'Integrated Pollution Control'** • Covers the discharge of certain substances to land, water or air • This area does not appear to have implications for imaging departments **'Duty of Care'** • The person disposing of waste should only transfer it to those who are authorised to receive it • Checks should be made that anyone receiving departmental waste, e.g. silver recovery firms, is licensed to dispose of the product
Water Act (1989)	• A trade effluent discharge consent is required • The amount charged is decided by the strength and volume of the effluent • Many economies (and some Water Authorities) set the silver level at 2 parts per million • The 23 most dangerous chemical pollutants are on what is referred to as the 'red list' • Silver appears on the next list (grey)
The Chemicals (Hazard Information and Packaging for Supply) Regulations 1994 (amended 1999) (CHIP)	These regulations cover such topics as: • The classification of dangerous substances • The symbols used for dangerous substances • The preparation of dangerous substances • Information for safety data sheets • The labelling of substances • The British and International Standards for child resistant fastenings and tactile warning devices The regulations are for manufacturers and suppliers • Hazard being defined as: 'the inherent properties of a chemical' • Risk: 'the probability of the hazardous properties of the chemical causing harm to people or the environment' The label provides information about the hazards and therefore the precautions which can be taken. These include: • Storage • Clothing to be worn during preparation • Correct handling • Disposal of material

(continued on next page)

LEGISLATIVE REQUIREMENTS FOR DEALING WITH THE USE AND DISPOSAL OF PHOTOGRAPHIC CHEMICALS ARE DEALT WITH UNDER THE FOLLOWING ACTS *continued*

Pollution Prevention and Control Act 1999 Implementing the European Council Pollution Prevention Directive (96/61/EC)	Follows the principle that the polluter pays and encourages the prevention of pollution. It is concerned with pollution into the air, water and the soil and covers both old and new buildings. Its aim is to integrate all existing legislation **Annex IV mentions:** • The use of low-waste technology • The use of less hazardous substances • Recovery and recycling • The nature, effect and volume of emissions • The reduction of the impact of emissions on the environment
European Packaging and Packaging Waste Directive 1994 (94/62/EC)	• Sets targets for the reuse and recycling of plastics, paper, cardboard, metal and glass • The target for packaging is that between 50 and 65% of waste should be recovered and up to 70% of commercial waste

ELECTROMAGNETIC SPECTRUM	
Range	Ranges from the low frequencies that are associated with radio waves, to high frequency cosmic rays 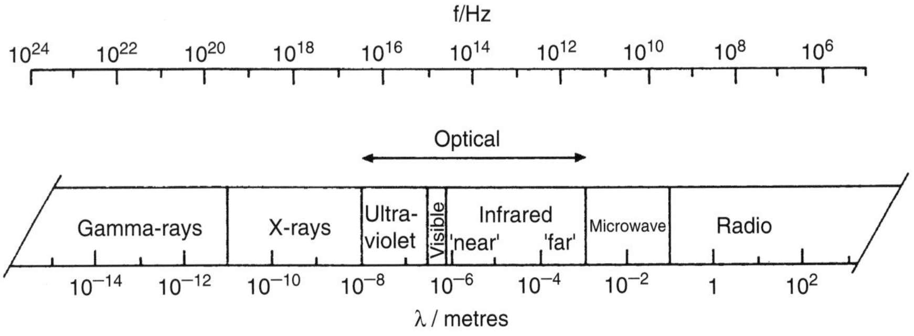 Fig. A.1 The electromagnetic spectrum.
Electromagnetic Radiation	**Wave theory** • Radiation consisting of waves of energy that are caused by the acceleration of charged particles • Consist of electric and magnetic fields that are propagated at right angles to each other and to the direction of propagation • In free space (i.e. a vacuum) they travel at a uniform velocity of 2.997925×10^8 m/s • Electromagnetic radiation depends on its frequency (f) and its velocity (c), the relationship being that: $$c = f\lambda \text{ (where } \lambda = \text{wavelength)}$$ 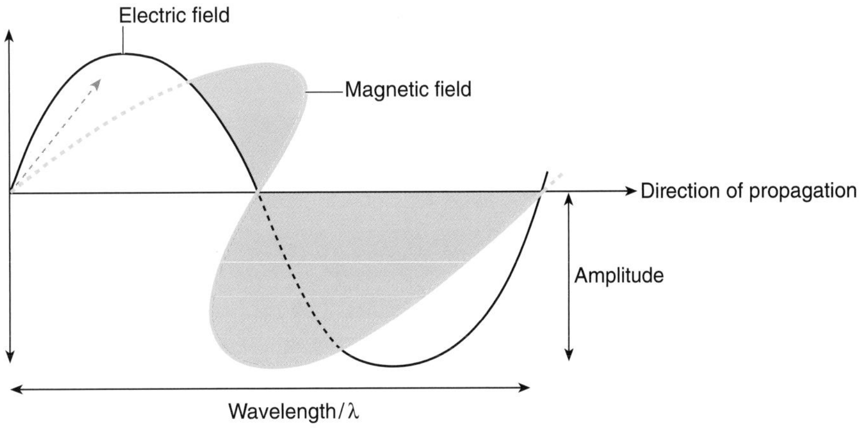 Fig. A.2 Electromagnetic radiation. **Particle theory** A stream of particles or quanta (photons) each having a discrete amount of energy $$E = hf$$ where: • E = energy • h = Planck's constant (6.626196×10^{-34} Js) • f = frequency of the radiation As velocity of the particle is constant, if the frequency of the radiation is doubled, the energy of the photon is also doubled
Visible Spectrum	400–700 nanometers (nm) and is a gradual change in colour from violet (400 nm) through to red (700 nm approx.)

Fig. A.1 The electromagnetic spectrum.

Fig. A.2 Electromagnetic radiation.

(continued on next page)

ELECTROMAGNETIC SPECTRUM *continued*

Visible Spectrum (*contd*)	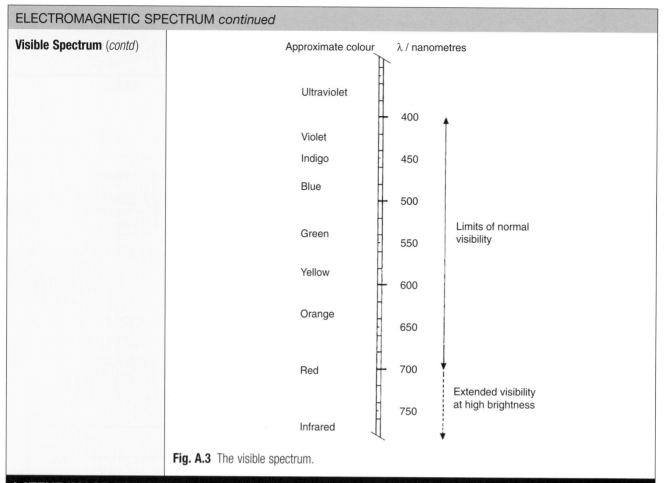

Fig. A.3 The visible spectrum.

LATENT IMAGE FORMATION

Definition	The image produced on the film after exposure but prior to development

MECHANISM

Emulsion and Silver Bromide	• Film emulsion is a suspension of silver bromide in gelatine • Silver bromide has a crystal structure (Fig. A.4) • Crystal grows with the addition of silver ions (Ag^+) and bromine ions (Br^-) • If the addition takes place in the light the emulsion dissociates and turns the emulsion black

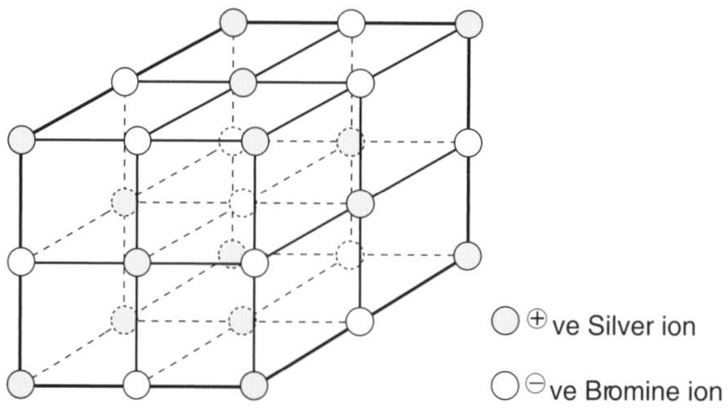

⊕ ve Silver ion

⊖ ve Bromine ion

Fig. A.4 Cubical silver bromide crystal lattice.

Gelatine	Has the following characteristics: • Chemical impurities, mainly sulphur, which produce 'active' areas in the silver bromide crystal • Physical defects in the crystal lattice structure which introduce electron traps • Growth medium, which allows silver bromide crystals to grow during the chemical reaction • Suspension and binding agent which is used to coat the emulsion onto the film base

(continued on next page)

MECHANISM *continued*

Electron Traps	Electron traps are within the crystal and are: • Areas of low energy that are caused by lattice defects and impurities (neutral colloids) from the gelatine • Where, after exposure, the latent image starts to form (Fig. A.5) 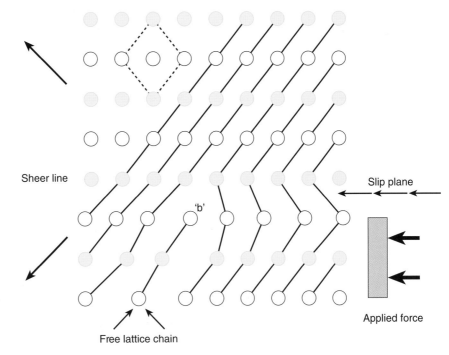 **Fig. A.5** Production of crystal lattice defects. **Note** There is an excess of potassium bromide used in the emulsion production. This: • Alters crystal shapes giving more electron traps • Increases the surface potential barrier of the crystal, thus improving selectivity (see Fig. D.3). Free interstitial silver ions are contained within the silver bromide crystal. They: • Provide the free silver that is necessary during the early stages of latent image formation • Balance the negatively charged bromine ion barrier making the silver bromide crystal electrically neutral
Effects of Exposure	Electrons released by exposure must be able to enter the conduction band of the silver bromide crystal 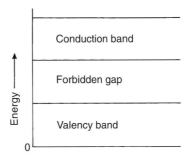 **Fig. A.6** Energy level diagram. **Valency band** • Contains the electrons in the outer layer of an atom and may or may not be full • Electrons can take part in ionic or covalent bonding • Can form bonds with other atoms to form compounds

(continued on next page)

MECHANISM *continued*	
Effects of Exposure *(contd)*	**Forbidden gap** • Electrons with sufficient energy pass through this band and become 'free electrons' within the crystal and form the latent image • Electrons with insufficient energy fall back into an orbit **Conduction band** • If an electron has sufficient energy to leave its atom it can exist in this band • The electron leaves a gap in a higher orbit called a 'hole' • The 'hole' is effectively a unit of positive charge

THEORIES OF LATENT IMAGE FORMATION

Gurney Mott Theory	**Nucleation**

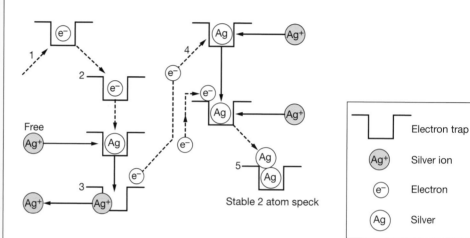

Fig. A.7 Diagrammatic representation of the Gurney Mott theory.

Stage one
• An electron that has been released by exposure is captured by a trapping centre and temporarily held
• A mobile, positively charged silver ion may migrate to this centre and form a silver atom, but . . .

Stage two
• The electron may escape from the trap due to its vibrational energy and again become free in the conduction band
• Eventually it becomes trapped long enough to be joined by a silver ion giving a silver atom

Stage three
• A single silver atom is unstable, separation occurs and stages one and two happen again

Stage four
• The single silver atom can act as a trap for another electron, and if another silver ion is attracted to this site

Stage five
• A stable two-atom silver speck is formed and is called a latent sub-image centre

Growth
• Electron trap deepens
• Free interstitial ions are attracted causing a build up of silver atoms
• The surface potential barrier of the crystal is broken making the crystal susceptible to development
• When growth is complete the centres are called development centres

(continued on next page)

THEORIES OF LATENT IMAGE FORMATION *continued*

Mitchell Theory	**Nucleation**

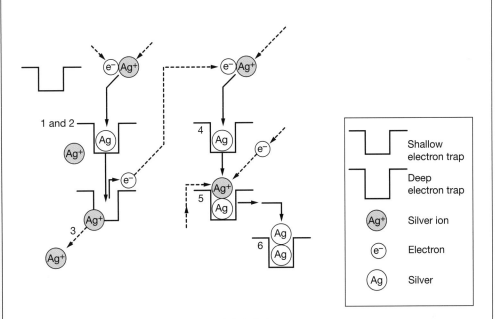

Fig. A.8 Diagrammatic representation of the Mitchell theory.

Stages one and two
- A free silver ion comes near to a shallow electron trap and deepens it
- While this trap is deepened, a free electron, released by exposure, and another free silver ion approach the trap together and immediately form a silver atom
- This is called a pre-image centre

Stage three
- The single silver atom is unstable and it dissociates into a silver ion and an electron

Stages four and five
- Stages one and two re-occur
- The single silver atom must acquire a second silver ion. If it is successful and an electron arrives before the escape of this second silver ion, a stable *latent sub-image centre* forms

Growth
- See Gurney Mott theory

STRUCTURE OF THE FILM EMULSION

	• The film emulsion is the basic 'sensitive material' used to record the image • It is a suspension of a suitable light-sensitive salt (i.e. the silver halides) within a gelatine binder • This suspension is coated on a supporting medium called the base • Is subject to other coatings in order to protect it from damage
Silver Halide	Silver bromide (AgBr) is the halide of choice, it is: • Not sensitive to wavelengths above 480 nm (cut off sensitivity) • Most sensitive to 430 nm, blue light (peak sensitivity) • Used with 2–4% silver bromide • Colour sensitisers (dyes) extend the spectral sensitivity

(continued on next page)

STRUCTURE OF THE FILM EMULSION *continued*

Silver Halide (*contd*)	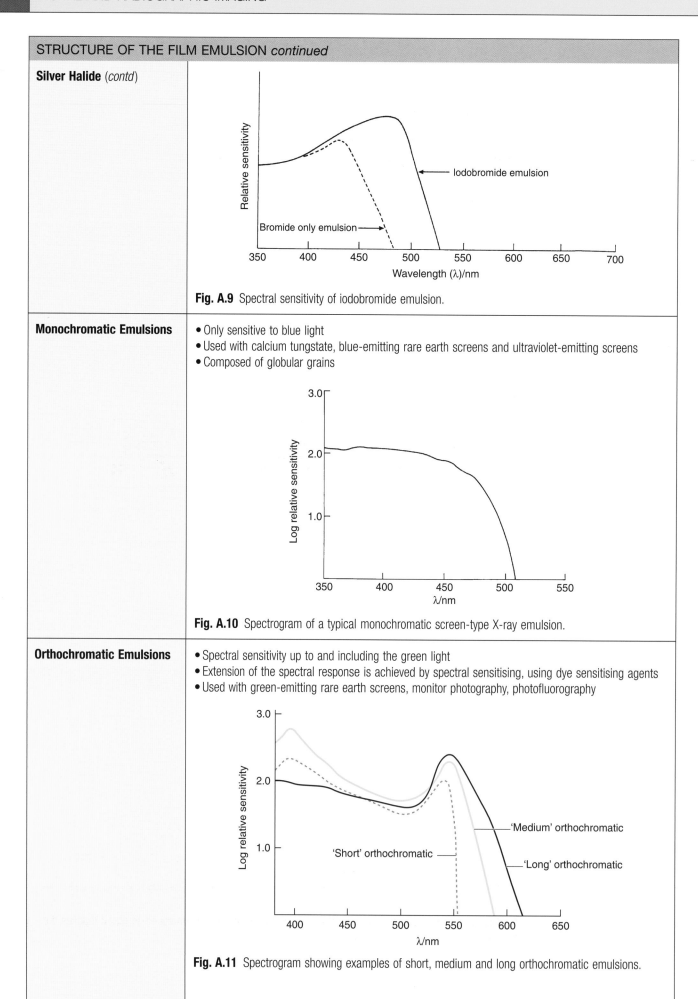

Fig. A.9 Spectral sensitivity of iodobromide emulsion.

Monochromatic Emulsions

- Only sensitive to blue light
- Used with calcium tungstate, blue-emitting rare earth screens and ultraviolet-emitting screens
- Composed of globular grains

Fig. A.10 Spectrogram of a typical monochromatic screen-type X-ray emulsion.

Orthochromatic Emulsions

- Spectral sensitivity up to and including the green light
- Extension of the spectral response is achieved by spectral sensitising, using dye sensitising agents
- Used with green-emitting rare earth screens, monitor photography, photofluorography

Fig. A.11 Spectrogram showing examples of short, medium and long orthochromatic emulsions.

GRAININESS	
Definition	Graininess is the perception of the apparent granular structure of the image
Properties	• Graininess in a radiograph is chiefly a product of *exposure* • Graininess impairs *perception of small details* far more than large details • The *contrast of details* must be higher on the film if significant graininess is present • The largest constituent of graininess on screen film is *quantum mottle* • Graininess reduces *image quality* and perceptibility Is influenced by: • The relatively coarse structure of the silver halide grains • Quantum mottle
Film Grain	Silver halide grains in the emulsion are of microscopic size When the latent image is formed, the alteration to the crystal is not visible, even under an electron microscope. It is only developer that can amplify this effect Developer + silver bromide = an amplification factor of 10^9 • After development, threads of metallic silver merge with the threads of neighbouring crystals causing visible graininess, which is increased due to the superimposition of the two emulsions The perfect system images the 'arrowhead' perfectly with no grain. D = 1.0 (a) A 'slow' system absorbs 20 quanta → 40 developed grains → D = 1.0 NB: Some definition of arrowhead is lost (b) A fast system. Film is now 2x the speed .˙. only 10 quanta must produce 4 developed grains per collision to reach D = 1.0. Even more definition is lost. The image is 'grainy' x = Quanta collision • = Developed grain **Fig. A.12** Diagrammatic illustration of film grain in relation to film speed. In general it can be said that: • The higher the speed of the film, the greater the inherent film grain • The diagram shows the effect of film grain • If a high speed radiographic film is exposed to *light*, grain is barely visible • It can therefore be assumed that the *largest significant factor* in the production of graininess is quantum mottle or screen mottle
Quantum Mottle Quantum mottle $= \dfrac{1}{\sqrt{\text{exposure}}}$	• In Figure A.13, high levels of irradiation result in the quanta being scattered fairly evenly over the film surface. Because of this high level of irradiation, the image can still be clearly seen • With half the exposure, only half the quanta are available (Fig. A.14). Now the image is not clear as the randomness of the quanta landing produces variations of density over the film • The dose is now so low that the film now begins to record individual quanta and the apparent 'grain' (the record of the single quanta) begins to appear • Exposures can be so low that only individual quanta will be recorded, insufficient even to record an image • Quantum mottle, therefore, has an effect similar to an increase of film speed, in that it reduces the ultimate definition of the system by increased graininess
	(continued on next page)

GRAININESS *continued*

Quantum Mottle (*contd*)

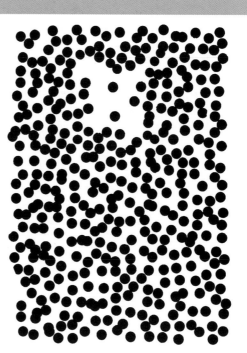

Fig. A.13 X-ray quanta striking film (representation of reality, with quanta striking film randomly).

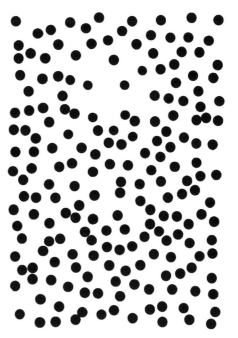

Fig. A.14 X-ray quanta striking film, half exposure of Fig. A.13.

GRAIN TECHNOLOGY

Globular Grains	Used in blue sensitive or monochromatic systems as the light-absorbing ability of the grain depends only on its volume. Globular grains have: • High volume • Good absorption • Good sharpness in relation to film speed **Fig. A.15** Diagrammatic representation of globular grains.
Tabular Grains	Tabular grains have: • A very large surface area but have a small volume • Very high resolution and relatively low silver coating weights, which produce a high speed emulsion **Fig. A.16** Diagrammatic representation of tabular grains. **Advantages** • Increased resolution; due to reduction in crossover • Reduction in silver coating weights by making the crystals thinner and flatter **Disadvantage** • Higher graininess; due to crossover
T-Mat™ Emulsions	• Nearly all the grains are identical and extremely flat • Resultant image is sharp but has an increase in graininess **Fig. A.17** Diagrammatic representation of (A) T-Mat emulsion, (B) T-Mat silver bromide grain.

(continued on next page)

GRAIN TECHNOLOGY *continued*

Structured Twin Emulsions	• The increase in the surface area of the crystal is achieved by using two tabular-type grains in combination • Resultant image is sharp but has an increase in graininess 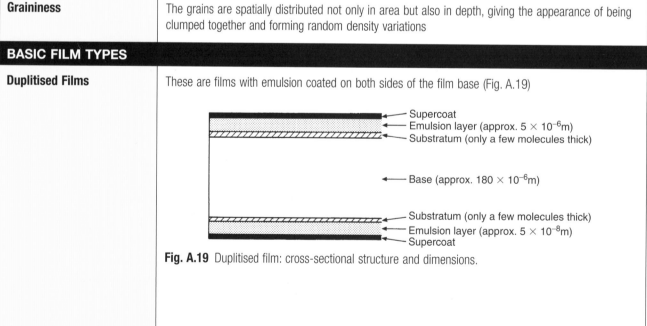 **Fig. A.18** Diagrammatic representation of (A) Structured twin tabular grains and (B) T-Mat tabular grains.

FILM TERMINOLOGY

Contrast	• Depends on grain size distribution (the range of grain sizes) • The larger crystals are most sensitive and the smaller crystals least sensitive to exposure
Speed	• Governed by its average grain size • The larger the average grain size the more sensitive the film and the greater its speed • Fast film tends towards low contrast and slower film towards high contrast
Graininess	The grains are spatially distributed not only in area but also in depth, giving the appearance of being clumped together and forming random density variations

BASIC FILM TYPES

Duplitised Films	These are films with emulsion coated on both sides of the film base (Fig. A.19) Supercoat Emulsion layer (approx. 5×10^{-6}m) Substratum (only a few molecules thick) Base (approx. 180×10^{-6}m) Substratum (only a few molecules thick) Emulsion layer (approx. 5×10^{-8}m) Supercoat **Fig. A.19** Duplitised film: cross-sectional structure and dimensions.

(continued on next page)

BASIC FILM TYPES *continued*	

Duplitised Films (*contd*)	**Advantages**
	• Increased film speed
	  ○ Reduces dose to the patient
	  ○ Reduces movement unsharpness (due to decreased exposure times)
	  ○ Reduces geometric unsharpness (e.g. if smaller focal spots are used)
	  ○ Reduces potential dose to staff
	• Increased contrast
	
	Disadvantage of duplitisation
	• Very slight increase in photographic unsharpness due to the parallax effect (Fig. A.20)
	
	Fig. A.20 Image distortion due to parallax.

The Base	Polyester (polyethylene terephthalate) **Blue base** • In continuous viewing, is much more restful on the viewer's eyes • Produces a slightly higher visual contrast than clear base • Gives a more aesthetically pleasing image **Clear base** • Has a very low base fog when compared to a blue-based film • The basic fog remains low even when viewed on poor viewing equipment • There is a slight increase in perceptibility in the toe of the curve due to the lower base fog, which makes this type of base suitable for ultrasound work • There is slightly lower visual contrast • Continued viewing of a clear-based film may be more tiresome for some viewers
Substratum	An adhesive layer that binds the emulsion to the base
Emulsion	• A mixture of gelatine and the silver bromide (silver halides of bromine) • The shapes of the crystals in this suspension may range from globular to tabular grains • There may be dye sensitising agents present in order to control the spectral sensitivity characteristics of the film
Supercoat	• This is a thin layer of clear, hardened gelatine coated onto the top surface of the emulsion • It protects the emulsion from mechanical damage

SCREEN-TYPE DUPLITISED FILMS

'Standard Contrast'-Type Emulsions	• Base + fog = 0.18 • Average gradient (G) = 2.6 • Maximum density (D max) = 3.5–4.0 • Speed = log It 1.53 (at net density 1.0). 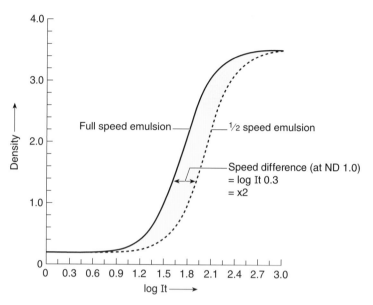 **Fig. A.21** Characteristic curves of conventional and 'half speed'-type emulsion.
Half Speed-type Emulsions	• Characteristics as for standard contrast but with half the speed • Improved image quality • Increased patient dose
Latitude or 'L'-type Emulsions	• Specifically introduced to improve the detail seen in the peripheral areas of chest radiography • Increased film latitude • At higher densities the gradient of the characteristic curve decreases • Average gradient = 2.2 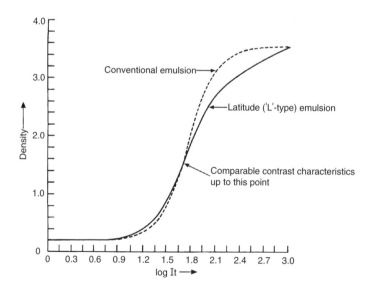 **Fig. A.22** Characteristic curve of a latitude ('L')-type emulsion (compared with a conventional emulsion).

OTHER DUPLITISED EMULSIONS

Split Emulsion Films	Designed specifically for mammography and have: • Protective top coating • Cubic crystal emulsion layer 1 of high contrast • Cubic crystal emulsion layer 2 to give high D max and contrast • Base • Antihalation layer • Protective top coating
Contrast or 'C' Type Emulsions	Designed for chest radiography and have: • A *very* low contrast • Mono- or orthochromatic emulsion • Fog and speed characteristics similar to standard contrast films • Wide grey scale rendition that makes the film appear to be lacking in detail
High Speed Emulsions	• High speed films. They produce (approximately) an 800 speed class when used with regular screens (this would be 200 with standard speed films) • Use advanced grain technology emulsions • High resolution at high speeds • Orthochromatic emulsions • Have higher contrast than their conventional counterparts

DIRECT EXPOSURE DUPLITISED FILMS

	• Structure is the same as screen-type duplitised films • Films usually come in their own individual envelope with no need to reload into a cassette • Used for intraoral dental work

SINGLE-COATED EMULSIONS

Structure	**Supercoat** • This is a thin layer of clear, hardened gelatine coated onto the top surface of the emulsion • It protects the emulsion from mechanical damage **Emulsion** • Lower silver coating weight than duplitised film • Sensitised to wavelengths above 510 nm (blue) **Substratum** • An adhesive layer that binds the emulsion to the base **Anti-curl anti-halation layer** • Prevents the film curling during processing • Allows the film to stay flat after processing • Coloured dye that absorbs reflected light and therefore reduces halation and is removed during processing 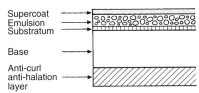 **Fig. A.23** Cross-section through a single-coated emulsion. *(continued on next page)*

SINGLE-COATED EMULSIONS *continued*

Halation	Caused by the reflection of light (which has already passed through the emulsion) at the boundary of the base with the air. If the angle of incidence is greater than the critical angle, the light may be reflected back and re-expose the emulsion layer. This produces a 'halo' unsharpness effect that reduces resolution. The density of the unsharp area is less than that of the true image 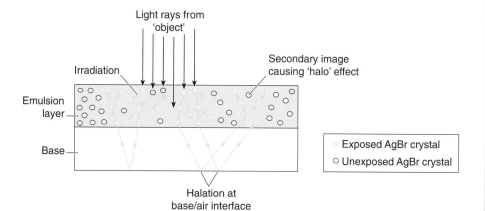 **Fig. A.24** Diagrammatic representation of halation and irradiation. **Identification of emulsion side** Achieved by the manufacturer cutting a small notch out of the edge of the film. When this notch is positioned in the top right or bottom left corner, the emulsion is facing the person handling the film

FILM FORMATS

Most Often-used Metric Film Sizes • 18 × 24 cm • 24 × 30 cm • 30 × 40 cm • 15 × 30 cm • 35.5 × 35.5 cm • 35.5 × 43 cm	Films are available in a vast array of sizes and different packaging to suit virtually all possible situations. In Europe, metric sizes are used almost exclusively while imperial sizes still predominate in the USA

FILMS FOR SPECIALISED USE

Dental Film	**Use** • Intra-oral work **Film type** • Direct exposure film, duplitised emulsion **Spectral sensitivity** • As conventional film **Film formats** • 5 × 7 cm, 3 × 4 cm, 2 × 3 cm **Special features** • Covered in a 'waterproof' packet, and some manufacturers package two films together to enable two films to be produced from one exposure • There is a raised 'dot' on the film to denote the tube side after the film has been processed
Copy or Duplicating Film	**Use** • Producing exact copies in terms of size and density reproduction, by direct contact printing **Film type** • Pre-solarised single-coated with anti-halo/anti-curl backing

(continued on next page)

FILMS FOR SPECIALISED USE *continued*

Copy or Duplicating Film (*contd*)	**Spectral sensitivity** • Monochromatic but with peak sensitivity in the ultraviolet region of the spectrum, in the order of 350 nm **Film formats** • Available as sheet film, usually in a whole range of sizes from 35×43 cm to 18×24 cm **Special features** • A pre-solarised film is unusual in that an increase in exposure received results in a decrease in density. The average gradient should be as close to 1 as possible, to ensure accurate reproduction of the 'object film's' density range
Monitor Photography	**Use** • Imaging the video output from CT, MRI, and ultrasound units and other similar modalities, usually via a multiformat or other camera system **Film type** • Single-coated with anti-halo/curl backing **Spectral sensitivity** • Short orthochromatic. Peak sensitivity in the order of 540 nm. Cut-off sensitivity in the order of 560 nm **Film formats** • 5 in $\times$ 4 in up to 35 cm $\times$ 43 cm, to suit imaging camera in use **Special features** • Available in blue or clear base and high or low contrast for use in ultrasound, etc.
Imaging Intensifier Photography and Photofluorography	**Use** • Recording the output phosphor of image intensifiers, especially those used for barium and associated techniques and mass mini-radiography **Film type** • Single-coated with anti-halo/anti-curl backing **Spectral sensitivity** • Short orthochromatic. Peak sensitivity 540 nm. Cut-off sensitivity in the order of 570 nm **Film formats** • Available as sheet film (100×100 mm) or roll film, 70 mm $\times$ 45 m; 90 mm $\times$ 30 m; 105 mm $\times$ 45 m **Special features** • Variable contrast to suit individual radiologist choice and stable reciprocity characteristics between 0.001 to 1.0 s exposure

INTENSIFYING SCREENS

	Advantages • Reducing the dose required for a particular examination • Resulting in shorter exposure times • Less movement unsharpness **Disadvantages** • Unsharpness problems due to screen structure
Screen Unsharpness	Is influenced by: • The phosphor type, thickness and grain size • The presence of an absorption/reflective layer • Dye in the phosphor binder or supercoat • Poor screen film contact will cause the scattering of light and therefore unsharpness **Note** • If a fast film/screen system is used to try and reduce movement unsharpness, the inherent screen unsharpness may be greater than the reduction in movement unsharpness • If longer exposure times are used, because of the use of lower speed screens, this could cause an increase in movement unsharpness Therefore a compromise must always be made
Screens Used	• Double screen technique, e.g. conventional radiography with duplitised X-ray film in a cassette • Single screen technique, e.g. mammography; usually in special cassette (e.g. vacuum cassette)

UNDERLYING PRINCIPLES

Reason for Use	• To reduce the amount of radiation received by the patient • Screens convert X-ray photons into visible light
Image	• Produced 95% by light and 5% by X-rays
Phosphor	• Metallic crystalline solids • With high atomic number elements • With an ionic structure • With a low incidence of free electrons
Absorption	In screens: • The incident X-ray photons are absorbed in the phosphor material, 95% by the photoelectric effect and 5% by the Compton effect • Secondary electrons are produced in relation to the exposure received **Fig. B.1** Summary of screen function.
Conversion	The energy available from the released electron is converted into light photons by either: • Fluorescence • Or phosphorescence

(continued on next page)

UNDERLYING PRINCIPLES *continued*

Emission	• Photons released by absorption and conversion leave the phosphor material and expose the film • Producing the latent image and, after processing, a density that is proportional to their intensity • The wavelength of the emissions is controlled in manufacture to match the peak sensitivity of the film it is exposing
Crystal Physics	• Crystalline solids comprise a regular three-dimensional array of atoms or molecules • The predominant bonding type is ionic bonding: this involves the transfer of electrons between atoms, resulting in positive and negative ions which then combine in a regular pattern to give a relatively stable configuration ● = ⊕ve Silver ion ○ = ⊖ve Bromine ion **Fig. B.2** Cubic crystal lattice: silver bromide.
Energy Levels	**Valence band** • The electrons are so loosely bound to their parent nucleus that they are free for sharing by adjacent atoms or molecules **Forbidden band** • Electrons within a system can only have a certain allowable range of energies • The forbidden band is the range of energies outside this allowable range • Electrons may 'pass through' this gap if they are energetic enough • But cannot exist in any form within this area **Conduction band** • Any electrons within this band are free to move providing they maintain a certain minimum energy • If they fall below this minimum, they return to the valence band or other vacant electron site • If a potential difference is applied to a substance with electrons in its conduction band, an electric current can be made to flow 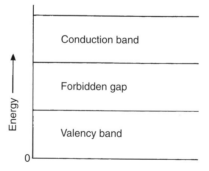 **Fig. B.3** Simplified energy level diagram.

(continued on next page)

UNDERLYING PRINCIPLES *continued*

Crystal Defects

Departures from the regularity of the ionic structure are called *defects*
- Point defects
  - Frenkel defect
  - Schottky defect

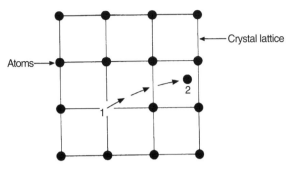

1. Vacant site
2. Interstitial ion/atom

Fig. B.4 Frenkel defect.

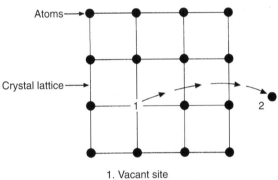

1. Vacant site
2. Atom out of position

Fig. B.5 Schottky defect.

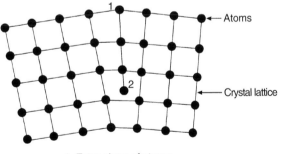

1. Extra plane of atoms
2. Dislocation extends into crystal

Fig. B.6 Edge dislocation defect.

- Line defects
  - Edge dislocations
  - Screw dislocation
- Create areas of 'low energy' within the crystal, called 'electron traps' and 'holes'
- The number of defects rises exponentially with temperature
- Typical values for point defects being 1 in 10^5 at 700°C for metals (i.e. 1 site in 100 000 is vacant)
- Defects can be produced by heating followed by rapid cooling, pressure and by ionising radiations

(continued on next page)

UNDERLYING PRINCIPLES *continued*

Crystal Defects (*contd*)

Traps
- These are areas of 'low energy' within the crystal that have the ability to catch and hold an electron for a period of time until it acquires the energy to escape
- The escape energy may be small (as in silver bromide) or very high (as in lithium fluoride)
- Traps are usually caused by two adjacent atoms attempting to share the charge of another atom, and are mainly the result of line-type defects

Holes
- A hole is the absence of an electron in the valence band; it is regarded as a mobile vacancy and has a positive electronic charge equal to that of a proton
- The 'hole' has the ability to attract an electron

Luminescence

Luminescence comprises two effects:
- Fluorescence
- Phosphorescence (or after-glow)

Fluorescence

- Light emission starts when the exciting radiation starts, and light emission virtually stops when the exciting radiation stops
- If the lag and continued emission is less than 10^{-8} seconds then the phosphor is said to fluoresce
- 10^{-8} seconds is used as this approximately corresponds to the time taken for an electron transition between energy levels to produce a light photon
- The incoming X-ray energy is absorbed, producing secondary electrons
- If the electrons have sufficient energy, they transit the forbidden band and become free in the conduction band. This leaves 'holes' in the valence band
- The 'holes' are immediately filled by electrons, either directly from the conduction band or from the electron traps within the forbidden band
- The transition results in another energy change that produces a light photon
- Any vacant trap in the forbidden band is now able to capture free electrons from the conduction band
- This does not produce a light photon, as the energy change is too small

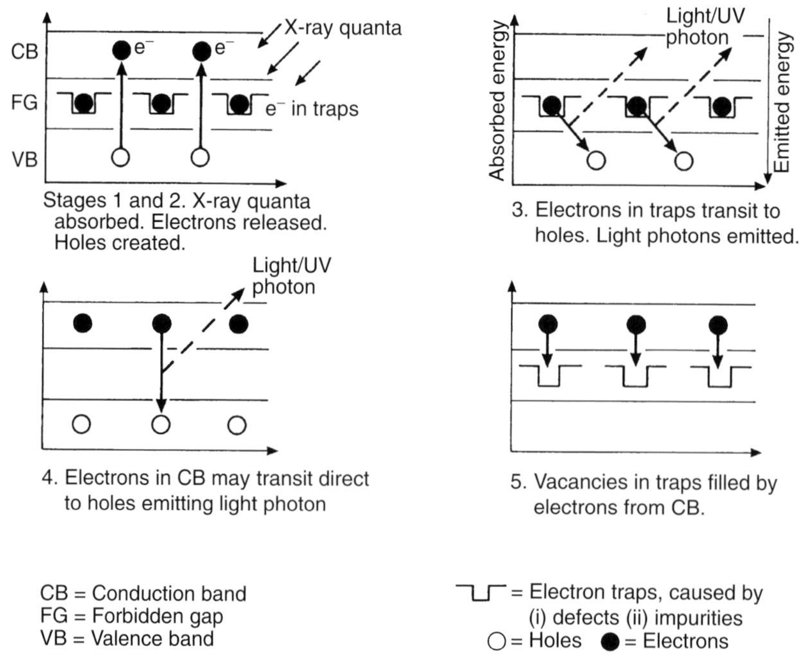
X-ray quanta
CB
FG
VB
e⁻
e⁻ in traps
Stages 1 and 2. X-ray quanta absorbed. Electrons released. Holes created.
Light/UV photon
Absorbed energy
Emitted energy
3. Electrons in traps transit to holes. Light photons emitted.
Light/UV photon
4. Electrons in CB may transit direct to holes emitting light photon
5. Vacancies in traps filled by electrons from CB.
CB = Conduction band
FG = Forbidden gap
VB = Valence band
= Electron traps, caused by (i) defects (ii) impurities
○ = Holes ● = Electrons

Fig. B.7 Fluorescence: diagrammatic representation.

(continued on next page)

UNDERLYING PRINCIPLES *continued*	

Phosphorescence or After-glow	• After-glow is the continuation of light emission even though the exciting radiation has stopped
	• If a phosphor takes longer than 10^{-8} seconds to reach peak emission or if it continues to emit light after this period it is considered to phosphoresce
	• The incoming X-ray is absorbed producing secondary electrons that, providing they possess sufficient energy, may become free in the conduction band
	• This creates 'holes' in the valence band
	• The free electrons then fall into traps where they are held for a period of time (determined by crystal type and inherent impurities)
	• If the trapped electron acquires enough energy it will escape from the trap and return to the holes in the valence band either directly or via the conduction band. In either case the energy change produces a light photon
	• The holding of the electron in a trap for a 'period of time' is the cause of the after-glow, as when the exciting radiation stops there will still be some electrons waiting to transit between bands
	• The length of delay in the emission is determined by the time taken for the electron to escape from its trap and return to a 'hole' in the valence band. This also determines how long light is emitted after excitation ceases
	• Phosphorescence in screens is an undesirable effect
	   ○ As it may cause multi-imaging
	   ○ And very occasionally film fogging
	
	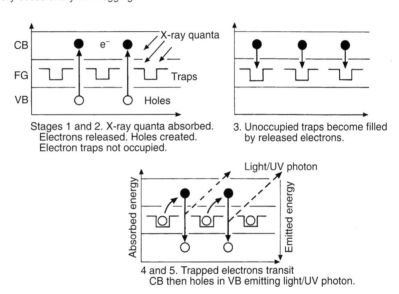
	
	Fig. B.8 Phosphorescence: diagrammatic representation (see Fig. B.7 for key to symbols).

Dopants	Impurities that are introduced into the phosphor crystal structure in order to control its characteristics. Dopants are normally one of two kinds: • Activators • Killers
Activators	• Impurities that stimulate the phosphor to emit light • The amount and type of activator controls the spectral emission of the phosphor to match the peak sensitivity of the film it is intended to expose • Lanthanum oxybromide (LaOBr) does not fluoresce unless it has a small percentage of activator present (usually terbium, Tb). Conventionally the activator is written after the main phosphor formula and following a full stop, e.g. terbium-activated lanthanum oxybromide is written LaOBr.Tb
Killers	Introduced to the phosphor structure to control the areas of the crystal responsible for phosphorescence and is therefore used to control after-glow

CONSTRUCTION OF SCREENS	
Base	• Polyester • No coloured tint • Base thickness varies but is approximately 250 μm • The reflective or absorptive layer is usually incorporated in the upper part of the base 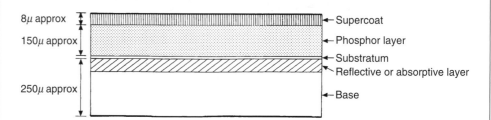 **Fig. B.9** Typical cross-sectional structure of a universal intensifying screen. All dimensions approximate.
Reflective or Absorptive Layer	**Reflective layer** • A thin coating (30 μ) of titanium dioxide (TiO_2) or similar compound • As phosphor crystals emit light in all directions, a significant proportion of that light is going away from the film • This layer redirects it towards the film, therefore ensuring that it contributes to exposure *Advantages* • Increasing the speed of the film/screen combination • A corresponding reduction in patient dose *Disadvantage* • Increases the amount of unsharpness produced **Absorptive layer** • Contains dyes • Light travelling away from the film is absorbed by a dye and does not contribute to the formation of the image *Advantage* • Improving the sharpness of the image *Disadvantage* • Slows down the speed of the system
Substratum	Used to attach the phosphor layer to the base
Phosphor Layer	• This is a suspension of the phosphor crystals within a suitable binder • It is approximately 150 μm thick • Acetate acrylate is used as the binding agent **Phosphor characteristics** • Even dispersion of the phosphor is required, as areas of high concentration would lead to uneven light emission from the screen and consequent uneven exposure of the film • Each phosphor crystal is surrounded by the binder • The coating weight is the amount of phosphor per unit volume • A screen with a high coating weight (i.e. a high amount of phosphor per unit volume) can be made thinner, and therefore produce a sharper image, than a screen with a lower coating weight in the same speed class • Light piping is a high phosphor to binder ratio. This enables more light to be emitted by the phosphor resulting in a sharper image being produced • Screen speed is determined in the phosphor layer; generally the thicker the phosphor the more light it will produce, and therefore the more exposure the film will receive for the same dose • Coloured dyes added to the binder can control speed and resolution without altering the phosphor thickness *(continued on next page)*

CONSTRUCTION OF SCREENS *continued*

Supercoat	A thin coating (about 8 μm) of cellulose acetobiturate, which: • Protects the phosphor layer from mechanical damage • Provides a surface that is easy to clean

INTENSIFYING FACTOR (IF)

$$IF = \frac{\text{Exposure required to produce ND 1.0 without screens}}{\text{Exposure required to produce ND 1.0 with screens}}$$

This is defined as the ratio of the exposure required to produce net density (ND) 1.0 without screens using a particular film, compared with the exposure required to produce net density 1.0 using screens with the same film

Effectively, the IF of a screen tells you by how much you can reduce the exposure required to produce a film if you put the same film in screens

Example

If a radiograph has been taken using a direct exposure technique, and the exposure required to produce an acceptable image was 50 kV, 25 mAs at 100 cm focus–film distance (ffd), what exposure factors would be required to achieve the same image if a screen/film combination with an IF5 was used?

$$5 = \frac{25}{\text{Exposure required using screens}}$$

Therefore the new exposure would be 5 mAs

Example

This technique also allows changes in exposure between two screens of known IF to be calculated, again providing the same film is used

If a screen/film combination with an IF of 10 was introduced into a department, replacing intensifying screens with a factor of 5, how would the exposure factors be changed to produce the equivalent image?

$$\text{Change to exposure factors} = \frac{\text{Original IF}}{\text{New IF}}$$

$$\text{Change to exposure facts} = \frac{5}{10} = 0.5$$

Therefore the mAs would be reduced by a factor of 0.5

Note

IF should be quoted at a particular kV value or range of values; this is because:
• Absorption of X-ray photons in the screen depends principally on the value, in photon energy, kiloelectron volts (keV), of the K absorption edge of the heavy element present in the phosphor
• The degree of photoelectric absorption will be high and, in general, the amount of light emitted will also be increased compared with the amount released by photons with a marginally higher or lower energy

Usually

• The higher the absorption
• The higher the light output
• The faster the screens and
• The higher the IF

When using calcium tungstate screens in the 60–90 kV range: an increase in exposure of 10 kV allows an approximate reduction in mAs of one-half, and will still produce a film of similar density
• i.e. 50 mAs, 70 kV is equal to 25 mAs, 80 kV in terms of film blackening

SCREEN SPEED AND DETAIL

Phosphor	N_t (Total efficiency) = N_a (Absorption efficiency) × N_c (Conversion efficiency) × N_e (Emission efficiency) Absorption efficiency = Quantum Detection Efficiency (QDE)
Phosphor Efficiency	• The higher the total efficiency of the phosphor the more light output • The rare earth phosphors gain an increase in overall efficiency by having a high absorption efficiency compared with that of calcium tungstate • The more efficient the phosphor, the thinner it can be coated to produce the same speed class and as a result the higher the image sharpness it will give
Thickness of Phosphor Layer	For the same phosphor type, the thicker the phosphor layer, the faster the screen but the greater the unsharpness it produces • If an incoming X-ray photon causes a phosphor crystal that is far away from the film to emit light • This light is given off in all directions but only some of it reaches the film • Therefore, the area of film exposed is larger than the phosphor crystal • This amount of spread of the light due to the distance it has travelled can be qualitatively expressed by the value 'U' • If the thickness of the phosphor is increased, the value of 'U' also increases and the unsharpness produced increases • However, if the phosphor is thicker, more of the incoming X-ray photons will be absorbed, the total efficiency will increase and more light photons will be given off. Consequently, to produce a similar film density a reduction in exposure will be required, i.e. the screen has increased in speed **Fig. B.10** Unsharpness due to screens: area of film exposed greater than that of the phosphor crystal. **Fig. B.11** Screen unsharpness: quantitative approach.
Coating Weight	This is the amount of phosphor present per unit volume. The higher the coating weight, the faster the screen • The more phosphor crystals there are in a given volume • The more light will be emitted

(continued on next page)

SCREEN SPEED AND DETAIL *continued*

Presence of Reflective Layer	• If the layer is reflective any light going away from the film is redirected towards the film and contributes to its exposure • The effective speed of the screen is increased but so is unsharpness • This is due to the internal reflection increasing the 'U' value **Fig. B.12** Screen unsharpness. (A) Thicker phosphor layer; (B) internal reflection.
Presence of Absorptive Layer	• The absorptive layer is a coloured dye that absorbs light going away from the film • This reduces the speed of the screen (because of the reduction in light reaching the film) and also reduces the degree of unsharpness
Presence of Dye in Phosphor Binder	• *The principal is covered by Beer–Lambert Law*, i.e. the greater the distance a ray of light travels in a coloured medium, the more it is absorbed • If a coloured dye is added to the binder, the value of 'U' decreases because the amount of light absorbed by the dye along path length ('x') is such that only a small fraction (or none at all) reaches and exposes the film • In order for sufficient light to reach the film to produce an appreciable image, the path length ('x') must decrease. This can only occur if angle α gets smaller and this in turn results in a reduction in the unsharpness ('U') • The dye reduces the exposure reaching the film. Therefore an increase in exposure is needed to obtain a similar film density **Fig. B.13** Screen unsharpness: reduction due to dye tinting phosphor layer.
Effect of kV on Speed	The rare earth phosphors are 'kV dependent'. In practice, this means that in order to make the best use of their total efficiency it is necessary to use them within a certain kV range, e.g. • System 3 has its maximum speed at approximately 90 kV (speed class 240) with quite a marked fall off at kVs higher and lower than this • If this system was used in a situation requiring a set kV of 70 kV, then its speed class will have fallen to 200

(continued on next page)

SCREEN SPEED AND DETAIL *continued*

Effect of kV on Speed (*contd*)	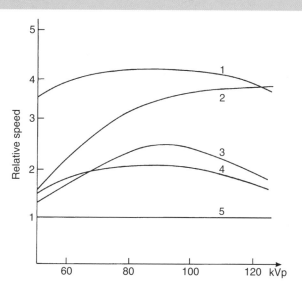 **Fig. B.14** System speed variation with kV. (1) A BaFCl.Eu system of speed class 350–400 (approx.). (2) A Gd2O2 S.Tb system of speed class 150–400 (approx.). (3) A Gd2O2 S.Tb system of speed class 130–240 (approx.). (4) A LaOBr.Tb system of speed class 150–200 (approx.). (5) A CaWO4 system (which is represented as a straight line for ease of comparison) of speed class 100.
Speed Classification	• Speed class is an easy comparison of systems in terms of speed (but not necessarily detail rendition) • It is based on an arbitrary scale with the value of 100 being the bench mark to which all other systems are compared • As the speed class goes up the amount of exposure required to produce an image goes down compared to lower speed class values **Speed classification: system basics** | Speed class	50	100	200	400	800
---	---	---	---	---	---
Required mAs[a] changes to produce similar densities (fixed kV + ffd)	200 mAs	100 mAs	50 mAs	25 mAs	12.5 mAs
Exposure alteration compared to class 100	×2	1	$\frac{1}{2}$	$\frac{1}{4}$	$\frac{1}{8}$	 [a]All mAs values are approximate.

SCREEN TERMINOLOGY

Crossover Effect	Crossover is the amount of light transmitted to the opposite side of the film base expressed as a percentage • Due to the use of duplitised film emulsions and multiscreen techniques • There is a decrease in image quality caused by the light, which is not completely absorbed in the first emulsion layer, passing through the base and exposing the second emulsion layer resulting in unsharpness • The widening light beam is the result of light diffusion within the grains as it passes from one side to the other, causing a 'wider', less sharp image in the emulsion layer furthest away from the initial light emission • The degree of crossover is usually expressed as a percentage, and varies from 15–25% in ultraviolet/blue systems to 60% in orthochromatic systems • Image degradation caused by 60% crossover is so great that it may necessitate the inclusion of an anti-halation layer as part of the film structure • In turn, this may mean that there is a requirement to use only a particular film with a particular screen in order to obtain the best results. This makes the film/screen combination a so-called 'closed system'

(continued on next page)

SCREEN TERMINOLOGY *continued*

Crossover Effect (*contd*)

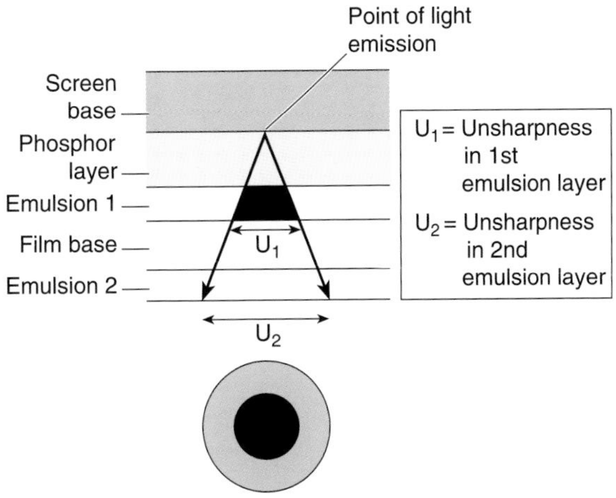

Fig. B.15 Crossover effect: showing unsharpness reduced in two emulsion layers.

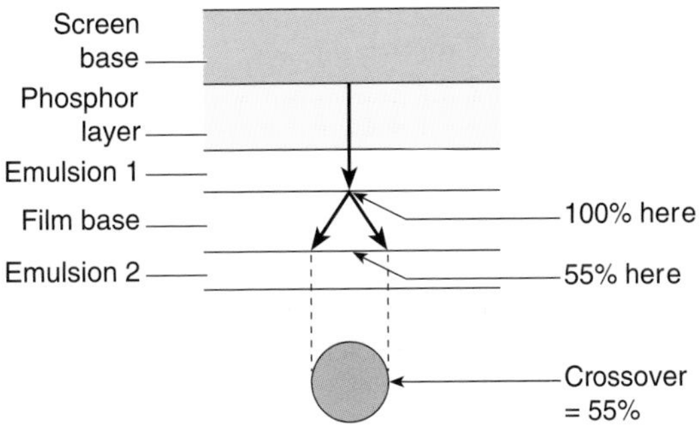

Fig. B.16 Crossover effect: calculation of percentage crossover. |
| **Resolution** | Measured in line pairs per millimetre (lp mm^{-1})
• A line pair is a line of a particular width followed by a space of the same width; so,
• If the quoted resolution for a particular system is 4 lp mm^{-1}, there are 4 lines and spaces contained within 1 mm, therefore each line is 0.125 mm wide and each space is 0.125 mm wide
• Resolution indicates the size of the smallest object that the system will record
• The smallest distance that must exist between two objects before they are seen as two separate objects |
| **Mottle** | This is the apparent 'granular' appearance in areas of apparently even density in the radiographic image
• Film grain
• Quantum mottle
• Structure mottle |

(continued on next page)

SCREEN TERMINOLOGY *continued*

Mottle (*contd*)

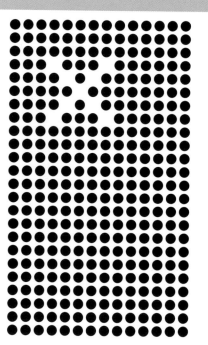

Fig. B.17 X-ray quanta striking film (theoretical representation).

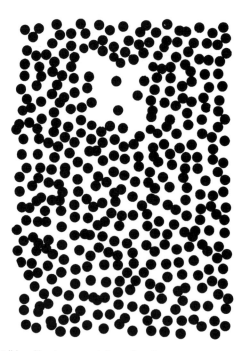

Fig. B.18 X-ray quanta striking film (representation of reality, with quanta striking film randomly).

(continued on next page)

SCREEN TERMINOLOGY *continued*

Mottle *(contd)*	 **Fig. B.19** X-ray quanta striking film, half exposure of Fig. B.18.
Film Grain	Film grain is due to the coarse structure of the silver crystals aggregating together (clumping) forming the overall density in the emulsion
Quantum Mottle (noise)	Quantum mottle is due to the random distribution of image-forming X-ray quanta producing non-uniform light emission from the screens
Structure Mottle	Structure mottle is caused by the fact that it is not possible to evenly disperse the phosphor crystals throughout the binder medium in an intensifying screen
Reciprocity	The reciprocity law states that: • The amount of density produced on a film is dependent only on the total amount of light energy employed • If the exposure (E) remains constant then the amount of density produced will also remain constant (all other factors being equal). Exposure is the product of Intensity I and time (t): $$E = It$$ • If the reciprocity law holds true then, providing E is constant, any combination of I and t may be used to produce the same density, e.g. if 100 'units' of E are required to produce a density of 1, then $$\begin{aligned} E &= It \\ 100 &= 10 \times 10 \\ &= 100 \times 1 \\ &= 1 \times 100 \\ &= 2 \times 50 \text{ etc.} \end{aligned}$$ All produce D = 1.0

(continued on next page)

SCREEN TERMINOLOGY *continued*

Reciprocity Failure	At very long or very short exposure times, the resulting density value was somewhat less than was expected • The use of very high mA and short exposure times, or • Very low mA and long exposure times ○ Will not produce the same result in terms of density as a set of exposure factors between the two extremes • Reciprocity failure seems at a minimum for times of 0.1 s and is so small as to be insignificant for exposure times between about 0.002 s and 3 s 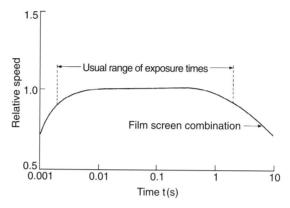 **Fig. B.20** Reciprocity failure: diagrammatic representation only.
Screen Asymmetry	In some intensifying screens: • The back screen may be slightly faster than the front to produce equal density on both sides of the film • If the two screens in a cassette are identical then the screen closest to the X-ray tube absorbs a proportion of the arriving X-ray beam and produces a certain amount of light • The back screen does not receive as many X-ray quanta, due to the fact some have already been absorbed, and therefore the amount of light output will be less • The front screen therefore produces a higher density on the film than the back screen • Therefore the back screen is made slightly faster, so that even though it receives fewer X-ray quanta its light output is the same as the front screen, thus producing the same density on both sides of the emulsion. This is normally achieved by the back screen having a slightly thicker coating of phosphor
Spectral Emission	**Matching spectral output** The wavelengths of light (i.e. the colours) that are emitted by the various screen phosphors. It is important to match the spectral output of the screen to the spectral sensitivity of the film. In general, failure to do this will result in a loss of system speed and a loss of information transfer from the emergent beam from the patient to the film <table><tr><td>*Phosphor name*</td><td>*Formula activator*</td><td>*Principal emission*</td></tr><tr><td>Lanthanum oxybromide</td><td>$LaOBr.Tb$</td><td>Blue</td></tr><tr><td>Gadolinium oxysulphide</td><td>$Gd_2O_2S.Tb$</td><td>Green</td></tr><tr><td>Barium fluorochloride</td><td>$BaFCl.Eu$</td><td>Ultraviolet</td></tr><tr><td>Calcium tungstate</td><td>$CaWO_4$</td><td>Blue</td></tr></table> Therefore: • Blue emitters are used with monochromatic ('blue') sensitive film and • Green emitters are used with orthochromatic ('green') sensitive film

(continued on next page)

SCREEN TERMINOLOGY *continued*

Kilovoltage Response	In order to obtain the best use of the speed offered by rare earth screens, the use of the appropriate kV factors is necessary

• Peak speed for rare earth systems are at 80–85 kVp, where speed is more or less constant
• With a fall in speed down to 60–65 kVp
and
• A sharp decline at kVp lower than 60

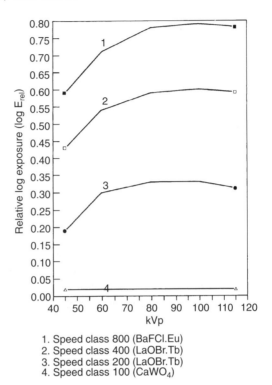

1. Speed class 800 (BaFCl.Eu)
2. Speed class 400 (LaOBr.Tb)
3. Speed class 200 (LaOBr.Tb)
4. Speed class 100 (CaWO$_4$)

Fig. B.21 kV response rare earth screens.

MANUAL PROCESSING VERSUS AUTOMATIC PROCESSING

Comparison	Manual	Automatic
Time	• Development 3–5 minutes • Rinse 10–20 seconds • Fixing 10 minutes • Wash 15 minutes • Dry 20 minutes Total 50 minutes (approx.)	• 22 seconds • – • 22 seconds • 22 seconds • 24 seconds Total 90 seconds
Economics	• Film hangers required • Manual movement of the film through the system • High water consumption • Separate room required	• Film hangers not required • Automatic loading and unloading of cassettes • Low water consumption • Space saving with daylight units • High initial cost of equipment
Factors	Variable times, temperature, agitation of chemicals and quality of solutions	Consistent times, temperature, agitation. Automatic replenishment therefore consistent quality of solutions

A TYPICAL AUTOMATIC PROCESSOR

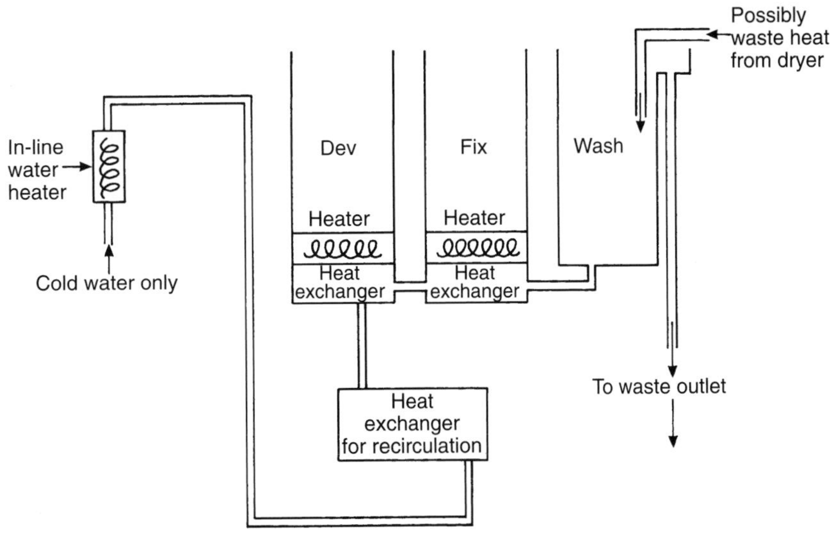

Fig. C.1 A typical cold water processor.

Film Entry System	**Construction**
	• Pair of rollers
	  ○ Grips film to take it into the machine
	• Microswitch
	  ○ Lies above the rollers
	  ○ Can be:
	    – An infrared light beam
	    – Trip wire
	    – Steady stream of air

(continued on next page)

A TYPICAL AUTOMATIC PROCESSOR *continued*

Film Entry System (*contd*)	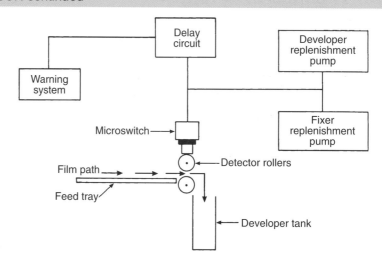
	
	Fig. C.2 Film entry system.
	
	Comments
	• Microswitch
	  ○ Activates a number of electrical systems
	• Replenishment
	  ○ The replenishment pumps are switched on when a film is between the entry rollers
	• Warning systems
	  ○ Can be by a bell, buzzer, safelight
	  ○ Indicates when it is safe to feed the next film into the machine

Transport System	• Formed by a number of rollers
	• Used to move the film through the processing tanks
	
	Hard rollers
	• Paper wound on stainless steel core and impregnated with epoxy resin
	  ○ Care is needed when cleaning hard rollers or the paper will be damaged and will then mark the films
	
	Soft rollers
	• Usually found between tanks
	• Constructed of a neoprene type substance
	• Motor turns the racks at a constant speed
	• Called 'squeegee rollers' as they squeeze the excess chemicals from the film before entering the next tank
	
	Guide plates
	• Made of stainless steel or plastic
	• Keep the film within the transport path
	  ○ Guide plates must be kept clean or they cause scratches on the films
	
	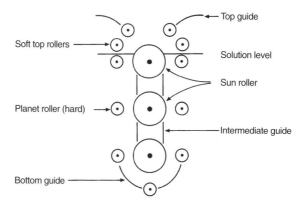
	
	Fig. C.3 Rack arrangement.

(continued on next page)

A TYPICAL AUTOMATIC PROCESSOR *continued*

Developer Circulation	**Thermostat**
	• Controls the temperature of the solution by switching the heater on and off
	
	Thermometer
	• Displays the developer temperature
	  ○ May be replaced by a light – when on the temperature is correct
	
	Heat exchanger
	• Linked to the water system
	• See water system
	
	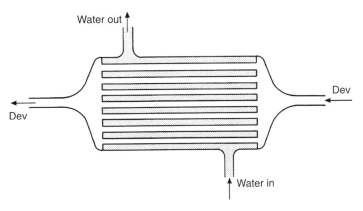
	Fig. C.4 Heat exchanger.
	
	Circulation pump
	• Circulates the developer
	  ○ Ideally developer from the bottom of the tank is reintroduced into the middle of the tank
	
	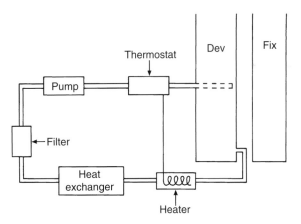
	Fig. C.5 Recirculation of developer.
	
	Heater
	• Maintains the temperature of the developer
	  ○ Developer passes over the unit that is linked to the thermostat
	
	Filter
	• Removes particles from the developer
	  ○ Stainless steel or plastic mesh

Developer Recycling	**Advantages** • Reduces consumption by 70% • Filtering can reduce the replenishment rate • Reduces the amount of waste **Disadvantages** • Additives may be required • Aerial oxidation reduced by using a layer of immiscible fluid on the surface of the developer *(continued on next page)*

A TYPICAL AUTOMATIC PROCESSOR *continued*

Fixer Circulation	• This is virtually identical to the developer recirculation • Oxidation is not a problem 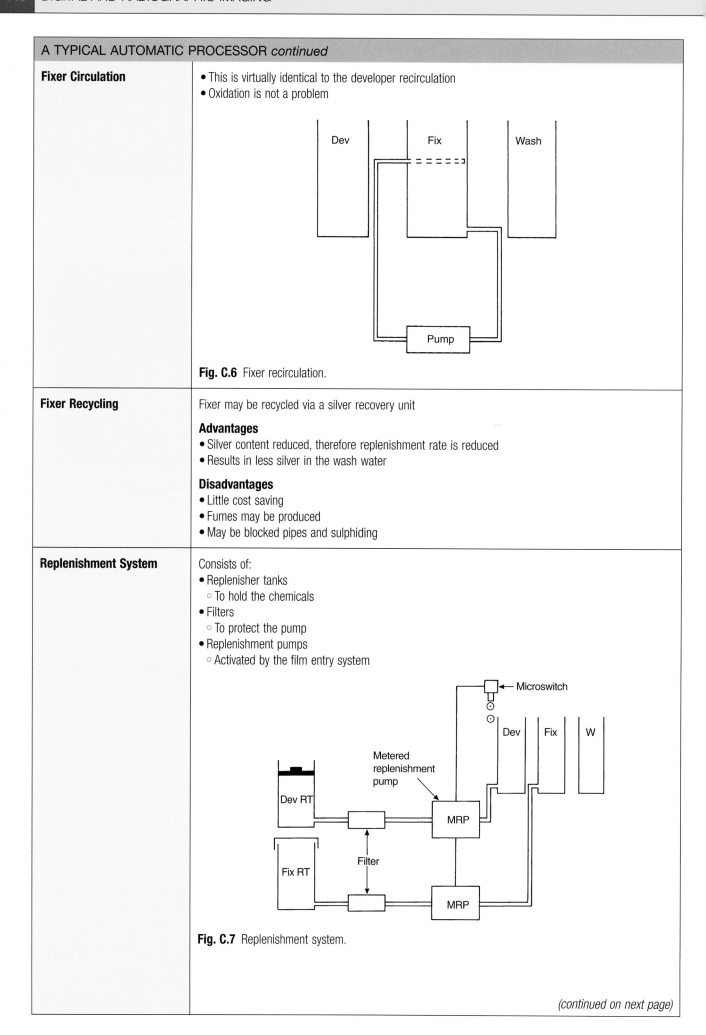 **Fig. C.6** Fixer recirculation.
Fixer Recycling	Fixer may be recycled via a silver recovery unit **Advantages** • Silver content reduced, therefore replenishment rate is reduced • Results in less silver in the wash water **Disadvantages** • Little cost saving • Fumes may be produced • May be blocked pipes and sulphiding

Replenishment System	Consists of:
	• Replenisher tanks
	  ○ To hold the chemicals
	• Filters
	  ○ To protect the pump
	• Replenishment pumps
	  ○ Activated by the film entry system
	
	Fig. C.7 Replenishment system.

(continued on next page)

A TYPICAL AUTOMATIC PROCESSOR *continued*

Water System	Consists of:
	• Hot and cold water supply
	  ◦ Ideally at 34 474 Newtons per m² (5 psi)
	• Filters
	  ◦ To avoid contamination
	• Mixing valve
	  ◦ Maintains temperature ± 0.5°C
	• Flow gauge
	  ◦ Indicates the rate of flow of the water
	• Temperature gauge
	  ◦ Gives operating temperature
	• Heat exchanger (see Fig C.4)
	  ◦ Box containing separate tubes, through which water and developer or fixer run
	  ◦ Water absorbs waste heat from the developer and therefore controls the developer temperature
	  ◦ If used for the fixer, heat is then absorbed from the water to heat the fixer
	• Maintains the wash temperature at least 3°C below the developer temperature
	
	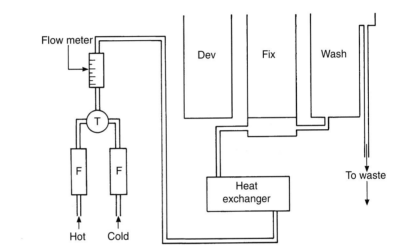
	Fig. C.8 Water system.
	
	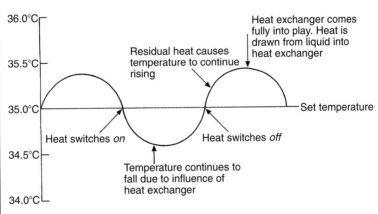
	Fig. C.9 Graph of thermostat response.

Dryer System	Consists of:
	• Roller transport system
	  ◦ Driven by the main processor drive shaft
	• Blower
	  ◦ Air flow to dry the films
	• Heater
	  ◦ Heats the blown air

(continued on next page)

A TYPICAL AUTOMATIC PROCESSOR *continued*

Dryer System (*contd*)	• Thermostat 　○ Sets temperature at 50°C • Filter 　○ To prevent dirt contaminating the films • 'Air knives' 　○ Increase the velocity of the air 　○ As air at a low velocity forced through a large diameter bore will increase in velocity if forced through a smaller diameter bore – Venturi effect 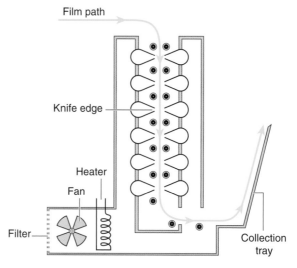 **Fig. C.10** Drying system.
Standby System	• The processor automatically shuts down if a film has not entered the processor for a predetermined length of time, e.g. 2 minutes 　○ Reduces running costs • Water supply – reduced to 5 litres per minute 　○ Maintains the developer temperature • Circulation pumps – developer left on, fixer shuts down • Transport system – stops 　○ Until a film is inserted into the machine and activates the microswitch • Dryer – stops
Microprocessor Control	Automatically monitors the following: • All solution levels • All solution temperatures • Dryer temperature • Area of film entering the processor 　○ Measurement by: 　　– Reed switches 　　– Microswitches *or* 　　– Infrared light 　○ To enable accurate replenishment • Transport speed

(continued on next page)

A TYPICAL AUTOMATIC PROCESSOR *continued*

Microprocessor Control *(contd)*	Width is measured by detectors Film Direction of travel Length is measured by various methods as described in the text Accurate measurement of area can then be made **Fig. C.11** Determining the area of film being processed.

DAYLIGHT SYSTEMS

	A film handling system capable of loading and unloading cassettes, without recourse to darkroom facilities
Advantages	• Better working conditions for staff • Better use of staff time, enabling more patient contact • Faster image production • Less opportunity for damage to cassettes or films • Fewer cassettes required due to the faster loading/unloading times
Dispersed System	Consists of: • Different sized magazines containing film • Film unloader for the cassette • Unloader is mounted on the automatic processor **Advantages** • More flexibility in the siting of equipment • Film dispensers and processors can be in separate areas • The film dispensers can be purchased in various sizes to suit the requirements of each work area • If a unit breaks down an alternative dispenser or film size can be used • The size of the darkroom can be reduced to save space **Disadvantages** • The initial cost of the system • The staff may have to walk further to process the films • Depending on the siting of the equipment there may be less efficient use of staff time
Centralised System	Consists of: • Film magazines • Film loading and unloading mechanism • Magazines and the loading and unloading mechanism are directly linked to the automatic processor **Advantages** • The system is quick to use • Loading and unloading take place in one place • The cassettes can be used with a conventional automatic processor • The size of the darkroom can be reduced thus saving space • In small departments the unit can be sited adjacent to the imaging room enabling the radiographer to maintain contact with the patient • There is no requirement for a dedicated darkroom technician, resulting in a better working environment for staff

(continued on next page)

DAYLIGHT SYSTEMS *continued*

Centralised System (*contd*)	**Disadvantages** • The initial cost of the system • If one part of the system breaks down the rest of the system cannot be used • If not correctly sited or the wrong number of units are purchased there may be work flow problems due to queuing at the unloaders
Microprocessors	Have been incorporated in daylight systems to: • Control the routine day-to-day running of the automatic processor in the daylight system • Keep a record of all film used • Monitor all service interventions • Record the electrical/electronic and mechanical state of the machine • Can communicate with external computers (notably the service engineer's) to produce a record and to run self test programmes • Have LED or LCD displays, giving details (for example) of faults occurring, size of cassette/film being used, etc. The film is either: • Automatically unloaded from a cassette via a light proof, spring loaded slot, the springs are opened by pressure on the unloader and the film falls down and is transferred into the automatic processor, or • A conventional cassette is used which is opened and the film is extracted by the use of suction pads and transferred to the automatic processor In a centralised system, the cassette is then reloaded with a correct-sized film. In the case of the decentralised system, the empty cassette is then taken to the correct-sized loader, where the film is automatically loaded into the cassette

PROCESSING FAULTS

Longitudinal Scratches	• Connected with the guide plates in the racks
Transverse Scratches	• Film handling in a darkroom
Pie Lines	• Chemicals drying on rollers ○ Line length equals the diameter of the roller causing the fault
White or Black Spots	• Roller damage ○ Caused by excessive cleaning
Drying Marks	• Dirt blocking the air knives ○ Only viewed by reflected light
Tacky Films	• Faulty fixation ○ Check pH and silver levels in the fixer

GENERAL FAULTS

Crescent Shaped Marks	• Poor film handling
Fingerprints	• Poor film handling
Static	• Dry atmosphere • Insertion/extraction of a film from a cassette ○ Screen cleaner has anti-static properties
Surface Marks	• Algae in the wash tank • Dirt in the tanks ○ Some processors automatically drain the wash tank if the processor is shut down

(continued on next page)

GENERAL FAULTS *continued*	
Pressure Marks	• Incorrect film storage ○ Films should be stored vertically

Radiation or Light Fogging	• Films irradiated while in the box
	  ○ Same mark on same sized films
	• Light leakage in the cassette
	  ○ Black mark round the edge of the film

Overall High Density	• Developer
	  ○ Fumes from developer cause fogging
	• Heat
	  ○ Temperature above 20°C
	• Storage time
	  ○ Check best before date on the box
	• Background radiation
	• Faulty safelights
	  ○ Check correct bulb (max 25 W) cracked filters

Sharply Defined White Marks	• Artefacts on or damaged intensifying screens
Milky White Stain	• Inadequate fixation ○ Under-replenishment of the fixer

The Concept of pH	• pH is a quantitative method of measuring the degree of acidity or alkalinity of a solution • The concentration of ions in a solution is indicated by the equilibrium constant: $$\text{Equilibrium constant} = \frac{\text{concentration of products in a chemical reaction}}{\text{concentration of reactants}}$$

pH Scale	• Ranges from 0–14
	  ○ Higher than 7 is alkali
	  ○ Lower than 7 is acid
	
	Note
	As this is a log scale small changes in value are large changes in ion concentration

Pure Water	• Pure water is chosen as the basis of the pH scale • It has its own equilibrium constant (Kw), which indicates the ion product of water • Kw constant has the value of 10^{-14} at 25°C, i.e. $Kw = [H^+][OH^-] = 10^{-14}$ • Normally it is slightly ionised into H^+ ions and OH^- ions • The acid portion of the solution is denoted by H^+ ion content and the alkaline portion by the OH^- ion content • Distilled water is neutral and therefore the ions are present in equal concentrations i.e. 10^{-7} mol/litre of each • To simplify the system the log of the reciprocal of the hydrogen ion concentration is used in practice

DEVELOPER

General Characteristics	• pH 9.6–10.6 • Can produce an image in the film emulsion in 20 seconds • Produces a maximum film density of 3.0–4.0
Conversion	• The developer must be able to precipitate metallic silver from the silver halide (silver bromide AgBr) in X-ray film emulsion Development $2AgBr$ + (hydroquinone) → $2Ag$ + (quinone) + $2HBr$ Reduction ——————→ Oxidation Silver bromide + Hydroquinone → Silver + Quinone + Hydrogen bromide **Fig. D.1** The chemical action of developer on silver bromide (simplified).
Selectivity	• The developer must be able to differentiate between exposed silver halide and unexposed silver halide • Changing only the exposed silver halide to black metallic silver • Selectivity ratio – the difference in rate between the development of exposed and unexposed grains of silver halide
Amplification Gain	• Amplification gain is a measure of the extent to which the developer increases the initial effect of exposure on the silver halide grains and is in the order of 10^9
Quality Developing	• Starter solution is added which contains a weak acid and bromide ions to initially suppress the activity of the developer • Developer replenisher + starter = machine tank developer • Replenisher is added when a film is processed to maintain the developer activity and is added proportional to area of film processed

DEVELOPER CONSTITUENTS

Component	Function	Comment
Developer Agent Phenidone hydroquinone (PQ) 1-phenyl 3-pyrazolidone and para-dihydroxybenzene	• High speed • Higher contrast than hydroquinone alone • Low auto-oxidation rate • Not excessively bromide ion dependent • Susceptible to pH variations • Temperature dependent • Superadditivity • Liquid concentrate • Less likely to cause dermatitis • Long shelf life	• Selective conversion of exposed silver bromide crystals (AgBr) to metallic silver • Possesses the feature of superadditivity ○ The combined activities of two developing agents in the same solution which is greater than the sum of their separate activities

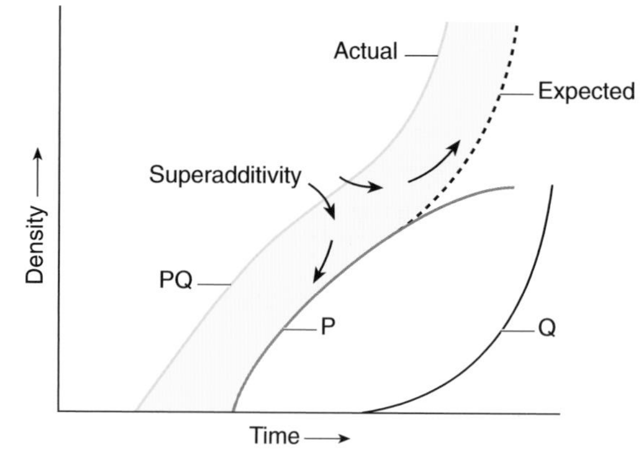

Fig. D.2 Diagrammatic representation of superadditivity.

Component	Function	Comment
Preservative Potassium metabisulphite	• Reduces oxidation to a minimum	• Caused by normal development action and aerial oxidation (exposure to air)
Accelerator Sodium or potassium hydroxide	• Gives the developer its pH value, therefore ensuring correct activity	• Accelerator is alkaline and ensures the correct image quality is given
Restrainer (anti-foggant) Benzotriazole	• Improves developer selectivity, between the exposed and unexposed silver bromide crystals, therefore reduces fog level • Also found in starter solution	• Increases the effective bromine ion barrier around silver bromide crystals • Has little or no effect on film speed • Gives high image contrast

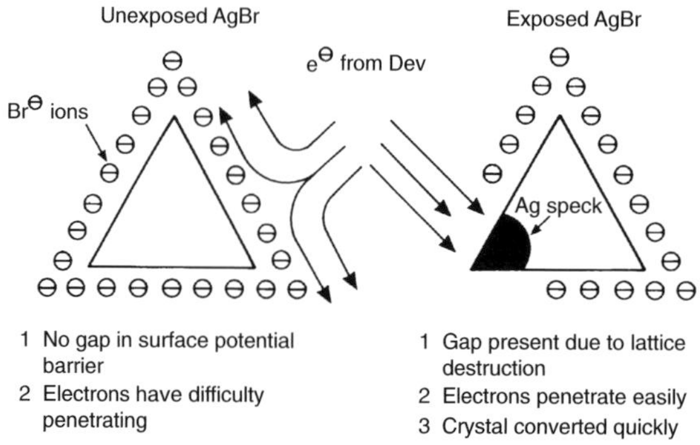

Fig. D.3 Effect of the bromine ion barrier.

(continued on next page)

DEVELOPER CONSTITUENTS *continued*

Restrainer (anti-foggant) *(contd)*	 Fig. D.4 The effect of restrainer on silver bromide crystals.

Component	Function	Comment
Buffer Boric acid + sodium hydroxide	• Absorbs the by-products of development • Therefore maintains pH within defined limits • And ensures that the activity of developer is constant	• Film development • Releases bromine ions from the film emulsion • And hydrogen ions from the developing agent • Forming hydrobromic acid which depresses the developer pH
Sequestering Agent EDTA sodium salt	• Softens hard water	• Changes calcium and magnesium salts into soluble complexes which do not precipitate out
Solvent Water	• Acts as solvent for all chemicals and by-products of developer action	• The use of plastic pipes prevents fogging of films from the absorption of copper from copper pipes • Filters remove grit and dirt from the water supply
Hardening Agent Aldehydes and sulphates	Reduces emulsion • Swelling • And softening	• Enables automatic processing • Prevents the film emulsion sticking to the processor rollers and being scratched or damaged
Wetting Agent Detergent-based derivative	• Reduces surface tension on the film • Allows even penetration of the developer	• Ensures uniform development of the film
Anti-frothant	• Prevents foaming due to reduced surface tension	Frothing and foaming is caused by: • Recirculation pumps • Replenishment pumps • The movement of the automatic processor rollers
Fungicide	• Reduces growth of fungi	Fungi formed • Due to the temperature in the processing tanks • On gelatin from the film

DEVELOPER CONSTITUENTS *continued*

Component	Function	Comment
Starter Solution Potassium bromide + acetic acid	• Depresses the pH • Adds bromide ions therefore restraining the activity of the developer on unexposed silver bromide grains	• Only required initially as the action of developer releases bromine ions from film emulsion into the developer solution

FIXER

General Characteristics	• pH 4.2–4.9, • If the pH is below 4.0 sulphurisation occurs • If above 5.0 white crystalline deposits of a precipitate of sodium aluminate are formed
Conversion	It must be able to: • Convert unexposed, undeveloped silver halide into a form that can be removed from the emulsion layer by the water present in the fixing bath, thus making the image permanent
Selectivity	The agent must have: • No effect on either the metallic silver in the developed image or the gelatine in which it is suspended
Quality Fixation	• During fixation there is a decrease in the level of the active ingredients in the solution and an increase in the level of by-products, resulting in an increase in soluble silver complexes and an increase in pH due to alkaline developer being carried into the fixer • Replenishment in the form of the addition of fixer solution and the removal of a quantity of used fixer solution which usually goes to silver recovery, see p. 159 • Replenisher is added when a film is processed to maintain the fixer activity and is added proportional to area of film processed (approximately twice that of developer) • Fixing time = 1.3 × clearing time where clearing time is the time taken for an unexposed area of film to become transparent

FIXER CONSTITUENTS

Component	Function	Comment
Fixing Agent Ammonium thiosulphate	• Conversion of undeveloped silver bromide (AgBr) into soluble silver complexes	• *Initial stage*: any developer is neutralised by the acidic fixer • *Stage one*: the fixer passes into the film emulsion • *Stage two*: silver sulphate in the film is changed to salt of silver ammonium thiosulphate (= clearing time) • *Stage three*: soluble silver ammonium dithiosulphate is formed which passes into the fixer solution

(continued on next page)

FIXER CONSTITUENTS *continued*

Fixing Agent (*contd*)	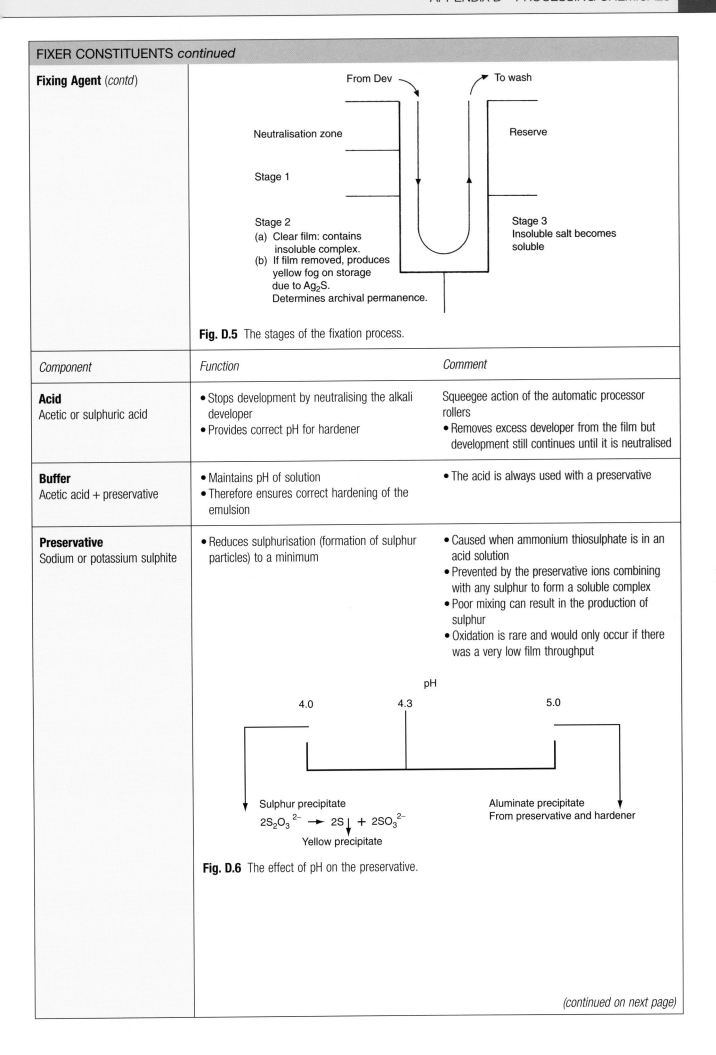

Fig. D.5 The stages of the fixation process.

Component	Function	Comment
Acid Acetic or sulphuric acid	• Stops development by neutralising the alkali developer • Provides correct pH for hardener	Squeegee action of the automatic processor rollers • Removes excess developer from the film but development still continues until it is neutralised
Buffer Acetic acid + preservative	• Maintains pH of solution • Therefore ensures correct hardening of the emulsion	• The acid is always used with a preservative
Preservative Sodium or potassium sulphite	• Reduces sulphurisation (formation of sulphur particles) to a minimum	• Caused when ammonium thiosulphate is in an acid solution • Prevented by the preservative ions combining with any sulphur to form a soluble complex • Poor mixing can result in the production of sulphur • Oxidation is rare and would only occur if there was a very low film throughput

pH

4.0   4.3   5.0

Sulphur precipitate
$$2S_2O_3{}^{2-} \longrightarrow 2S\downarrow + 2SO_3{}^{2-}$$
Yellow precipitate

Aluminate precipitate
From preservative and hardener

Fig. D.6 The effect of pH on the preservative.

(continued on next page)

FIXER CONSTITUENTS *continued*

Preservative *(contd)*

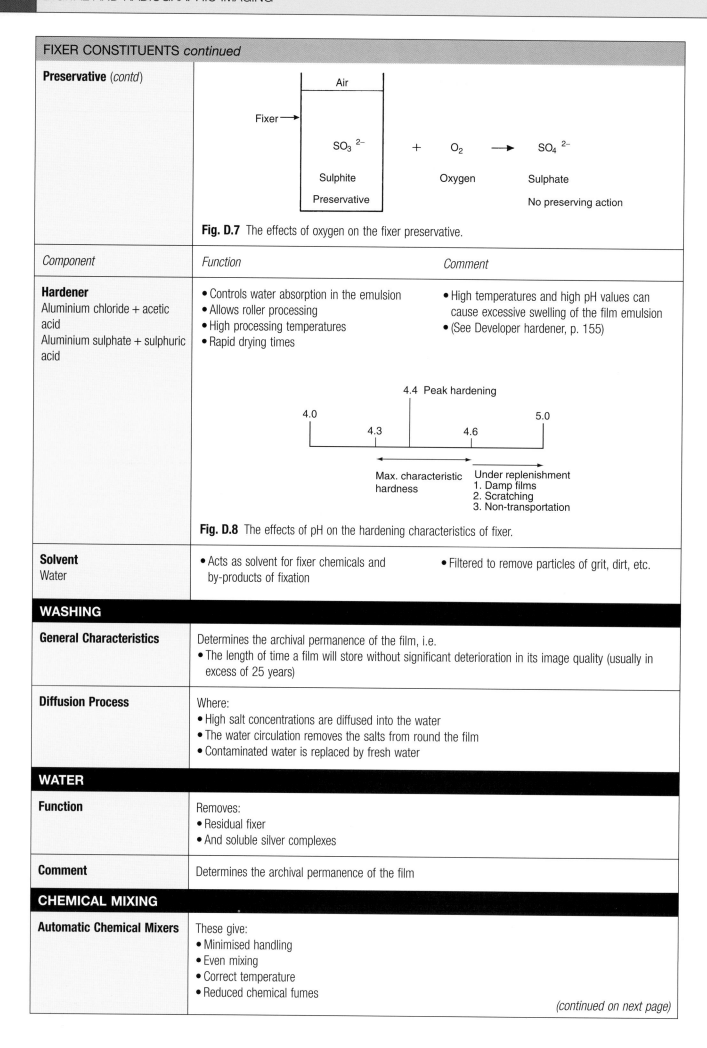

Fig. D.7 The effects of oxygen on the fixer preservative.

Component	Function	Comment
Hardener Aluminium chloride + acetic acid Aluminium sulphate + sulphuric acid	• Controls water absorption in the emulsion • Allows roller processing • High processing temperatures • Rapid drying times	• High temperatures and high pH values can cause excessive swelling of the film emulsion • (See Developer hardener, p. 155)

Fig. D.8 The effects of pH on the hardening characteristics of fixer.

Component	Function	Comment
Solvent Water	• Acts as solvent for fixer chemicals and by-products of fixation	• Filtered to remove particles of grit, dirt, etc.

WASHING

General Characteristics	Determines the archival permanence of the film, i.e. • The length of time a film will store without significant deterioration in its image quality (usually in excess of 25 years)
Diffusion Process	Where: • High salt concentrations are diffused into the water • The water circulation removes the salts from round the film • Contaminated water is replaced by fresh water

WATER

Function	Removes: • Residual fixer • And soluble silver complexes
Comment	Determines the archival permanence of the film

CHEMICAL MIXING

Automatic Chemical Mixers	These give: • Minimised handling • Even mixing • Correct temperature • Reduced chemical fumes

(continued on next page)

CHEMICAL MIXING *continued*

Manual Chemical Mixing	The operator must: • Use protective clothing • Mix in a well ventilated room • Mix in the correct order or precipitation will occur • Stir the chemicals well

SILVER CONSERVATION

	Silver is present in used fixer and films	
Method	*Process*	*Comment*
Collection of Used Fixer	Fixer collected by an external company	Reputable companies must be used that comply with environmental protection legislation
Metal Exchange	• Fixer is filtered through 5 kg steel wool cartridge • The base metal is replaced by the silver (5–15 kg of silver can be collected) • The metal ions are released into solution • The sludge is collected and refined	• Unit must be kept in a well ventilated area • Cartridge must be below the level of the fixer to reduce oxidation • Fixer flow must be at the correct speed • Output should be monitored by computer to ensure no silver remains (silver estimating papers can be used for a manual check) 1 gram/litre is the maximum acceptable level • Several units can be fitted in tandem • Unit usually runs at 70% efficiency

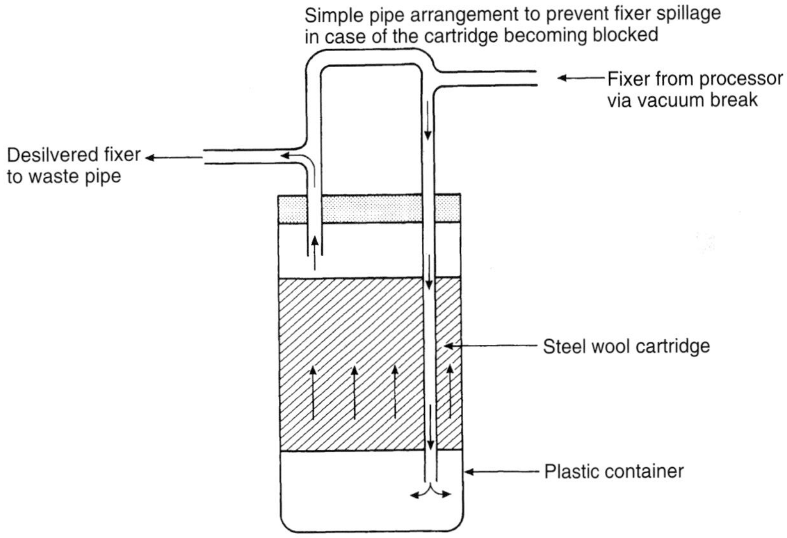

Simple pipe arrangement to prevent fixer spillage in case of the cartridge becoming blocked

Fixer from processor via vacuum break

Desilvered fixer to waste pipe

Steel wool cartridge

Plastic container

Fig. D.9 Diagrammatic cross-section of metal (ion) exchange in the silver recovery unit.

Electrolytic Recovery	Principle • Carbon anode and a stainless steel cathode are placed in fixer solution • A direct current is passed between • Positively charged silver ions (Ag^+) are attracted to the cathode where they are plated out as metallic silver	• Method produces very pure silver (95–98%) • Fixer can be reused • If the current is increased silver is deposited more quickly • If the current is too high or silver concentration too low, sulphiding occurs

(continued on next page)

SILVER CONSERVATION *continued*		
Method	*Process*	*Comment*
Low Current Density	• Originally used in fixer tanks of manual processing units • Used in conjunction with automatic processors with low film throughput	• Used when high current density units would be uneconomic

High Current Density	• Agitation of the fixer either uses:
	  ○ A rotating cathode/or anode
	  ○ A separate stirring device
	  ○ Or air being bubbled through the solution to ensure fresh fixer is in contact to prevent sulphiding
	• Microprocessors
	  ○ Monitor silver concentration
	  ○ Adjust current to give maximum return
	  ○ Indicate amount of silver being recovered
	  ○ And when cathode needs changing
		• Units can be connected in tandem, or
		  ○ one unit can serve several processors

Recover Directly	• Unit plumbed into processor fixer tank	• Usual to have an additional metal exchange unit attached to the outlet
Collection of Old Films	• Films collected by a specialist company	• Companies offer a price per kilogram • Credit against the assayed value of silver minus the service cost of the company

DEFINITIONS

Topic	Information	Comment
Density	The amount of blackening on a film • In Figure E.1 a light source is reduced in intensity as it passes through a film • Incident light = the light from the light source • Transmitted light = light passing through the film and observed by the viewer	**Note** No material is completely transparent

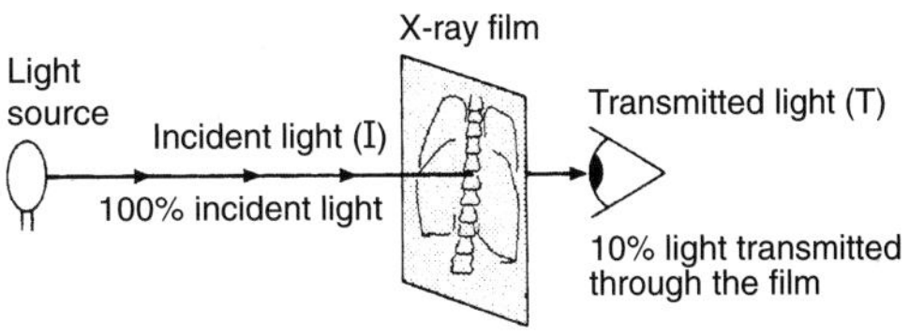

Light source — Incident light (I) — 100% incident light — X-ray film — Transmitted light (T) — 10% light transmitted through the film

Opacity	=	$\dfrac{\text{Incident light}}{\text{Transmitted light}}$	= $\dfrac{I}{T}$	= $\dfrac{100}{10}$	= 10
Density	=	$\log_{10}$ of opacity (i.e. $\log_{10}$ of 10)	= 1	(i.e. the log of the reciprocal of transmission ratio)	

Fig. E.1 Determining density.

Topic	Information	Comment
Opacity	I/T = 100/10 = 10 = opacity Opacity is always greater than one	I = incident light T = transmitted light
Log Values	Take the value of 10 for opacity The log value of 10 = 1.0 Therefore: Density is the log of the opacity	The log value 1.0 is the density of film when the opacity is 10
	• Film blackening is directly related to the weight of silver in the image • At density 2, only 1% of the incident light reaches the viewer • The density always increases with an increase in exposure factors • Because density is measured on a logarithmic scale it is easy to manipulate mathematically	• The blacker the film, the greater the silver content • Therefore 99% of the light is absorbed by the film • The exception is when solarisation occurs, see p. 169 • Density 1 plus density 1 = density 2

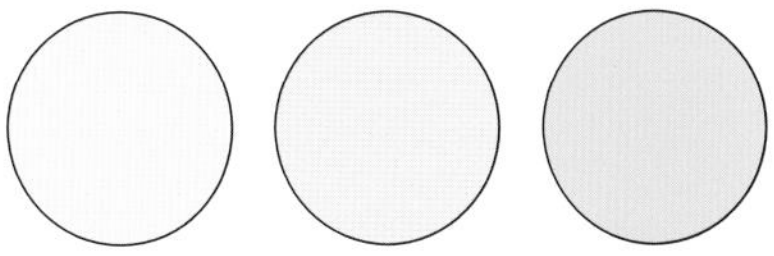

	1	2	3
Transmission	10%	1%	0.1%
Opacity	10	100	1000
Silver weight	X	2X	3X

Fig. E.2 Density is the relationship of silver weight, transmission and opacity.

(continued on next page)

DEFINITIONS *continued*

Topic	Information	Comment

The Characteristic Curve	**Used:**
	• To compare different *types of film*
	• To compare different *types of screens*
	• As a useful tool for setting up *exposure devices*
	• To determine *average gradient*, and therefore subject contrast amplification
	• To find film and exposure latitude
	• To find the absolute value of the *speed of films*
	• To monitor the performance of an automatic processor
		• A characteristic curve is a graphical representation of film density plotted against the logarithmic value of the exposure
		• The characteristic curve is also known as:
		  ○ A D log E curve
		  ○ An H and D curve (after Hurter and Driffield)
		  ○ A log I/T curve

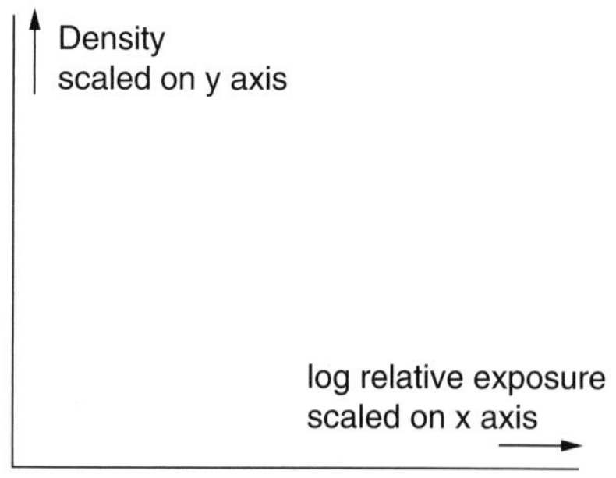

Density scaled on y axis

log relative exposure scaled on x axis

Fig. E.3 Establishing axes for characteristic curve.

PRODUCING THE CHARACTERISTIC CURVE

Name	Method of production	Comment
Time Scale Sensitometry	• The kV, mA and distance are kept constant and the exposure time is varied, always by a factor of 2 • By covering the cassette with lead rubber and exposing it section by section **Note** The first part exposed will receive the most exposure, the last part, the least. Eleven exposures are sufficient to plot a reasonable graph, although 21 would be better	**Advantages** • It is possible to process films at a known time interval after the test and therefore prevent varying latent image problems **Disadvantages** • The test is time-consuming to perform
Calibrated Step Wedge	• The use of an aluminium step wedge which has been calibrated in a specific way • The wedge should have a layer of copper on the base to help create a more homogeneous beam	**Advantages** • The step wedge can be made with any number of steps and as long as accuracy has been observed in the specification and manufacture an accurate characteristic curve will be produced • The step wedge can be reused • It can be used with different screen film combinations • It is possible to process films at a known time interval after the test and therefore prevent varying latent image problems **Disadvantages** • Because of the stringent specifications, a large calibrated step wedge can be initially, expensive

(continued on next page)

PRODUCING THE CHARACTERISTIC CURVE *continued*

Name	Method of production	Comment
Sensitometer	• A sensitometer is an exposure device which prints a pre-exposed negative directly onto the film • Care must be taken that the light output of the sensitometer matches the spectral sensitivity of the film	**Advantages** • Quick and easy to use • It can be used with different screen film combinations **Disadvantages** • The initial cost of the equipment is expensive
Pre-exposed Step Wedge Films	• Provided by the manufacturers • There are three common types of grey scale (or photographic step wedge) produced. They are: ○ The three patch wedge ○ An 11 step wedge ○ A 21 step wedge. Usually referred to as a root 2 wedge (Fig. E.4)	**Advantages** • Quick and easy to use • The films receive a constant, pre-determined exposure • The 21 step wedge gives the best results as it is possible to produce a better curve **Disadvantages** • The cost of the films • The films have a short shelf life • Can only be used to test processor consistency

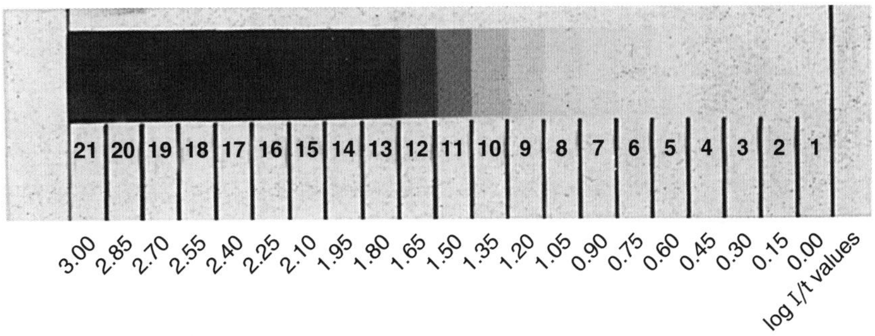

Fig. E.4 Typical sensitometer-produced 21 step wedge.

Name	Method of production	Comment
Densitometers	• Densitometers read the relative density of the various steps on the film by measuring the quantity of light which passes through an area • The more light that passes through the lower the density	• Information can be directly read off the LED display for each step • Then the characteristic curve is plotted by hand *Or* • The densitometer can be linked to a computer • All the steps are automatically read and the quality control information can be automatically printed along with the characteristic curve for the film • Information can be stored and weekly or monthly printouts produced to show the trends in processor activity and to allow comparisons between various processors

INFORMATION FROM THE CHARACTERISTIC CURVE

Densitometers (*contd*)	• From 0 to point 1, *Basic Fog* • Point A, *Threshold* • From A to B, The *Toe* • From point B to C, *The Straight Line Portion* • The area around D, *The Shoulder* • Point E, *Maximum Density* • From F onwards, *The Region Of Solarisation* 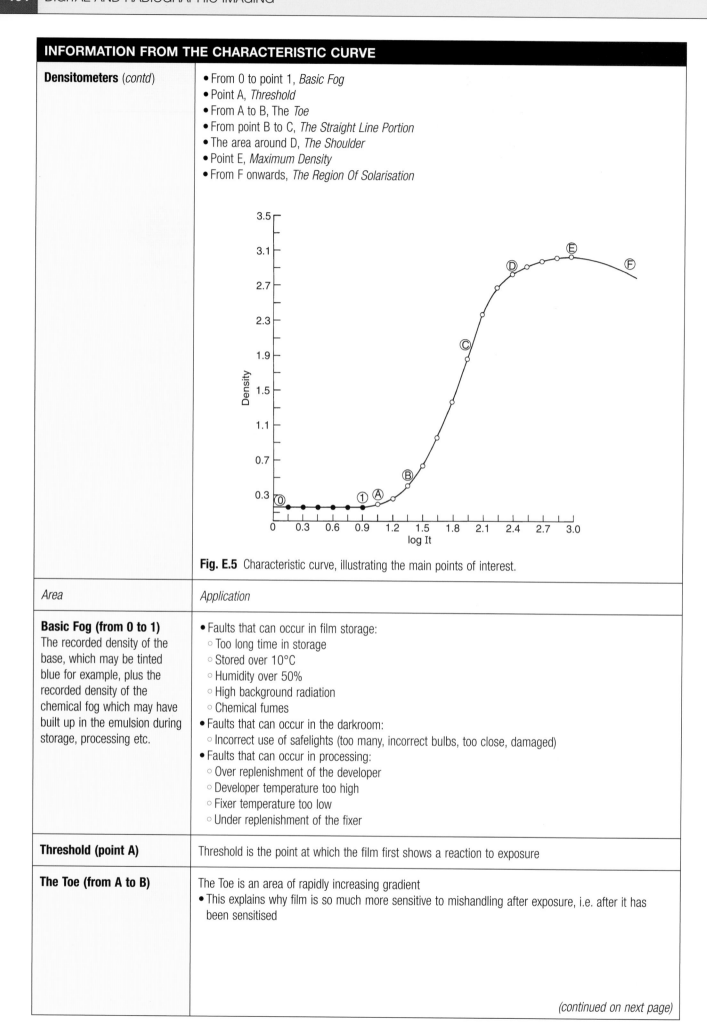 **Fig. E.5** Characteristic curve, illustrating the main points of interest.

Area	*Application*

Basic Fog (from 0 to 1)
The recorded density of the base, which may be tinted blue for example, plus the recorded density of the chemical fog which may have built up in the emulsion during storage, processing etc.
	• Faults that can occur in film storage:
	  ○ Too long time in storage
	  ○ Stored over 10°C
	  ○ Humidity over 50%
	  ○ High background radiation
	  ○ Chemical fumes
	• Faults that can occur in the darkroom:
	  ○ Incorrect use of safelights (too many, incorrect bulbs, too close, damaged)
	• Faults that can occur in processing:
	  ○ Over replenishment of the developer
	  ○ Developer temperature too high
	  ○ Fixer temperature too low
	  ○ Under replenishment of the fixer

Threshold (point A)	Threshold is the point at which the film first shows a reaction to exposure
The Toe (from A to B)	The Toe is an area of rapidly increasing gradient • This explains why film is so much more sensitive to mishandling after exposure, i.e. after it has been sensitised

(continued on next page)

INFORMATION FROM THE CHARACTERISTIC CURVE *continued*

The Straight Line Portion (from B to C) When looking closely at the curve (see Fig. E.5) it can be seen that there is no 'straight line' portion. The curve on medical X-ray screen film resembles more of an elongated 'S'	Used to determine: • Gamma • Contrast • Average gradient • Useful exposure range • Useful density range • Film latitude • Speed
Gamma	A measure of the angle of the slope–tangent angle A $$\text{Opposite/Adjacent} = \frac{\text{Side y}}{\text{Side x}} = \text{Tangent of angle A}$$ **Fig. E.6** Determining gamma.
Contrast	• The higher the gamma, the steeper the slope, the larger the angle, the higher the contrast (more black and white) • The lower the gamma, the less steep the slope, the smaller the angle, the lower the contrast (more shades of grey) • Therefore gamma gives the average value of contrast available in the image
Average Gradient (or average gamma, G)	Determined as for gamma but the line is drawn between net density 0.25 and net density 2.0 to give the average contrast • Net density = the density required plus basic fog • 0.25 – above this point variations in contrast can be seen • 2.0 – above this point variations in contrast cannot be seen due to the density of the image

(continued on next page)

INFORMATION FROM THE CHARACTERISTIC CURVE *continued*

Average Gradient (or average gamma, G) (contd)	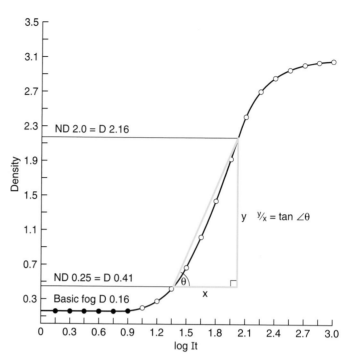 **Fig. E.7** Determining average gradient (G).
Final Contrast	Image contrast = subject contrast × average gradient 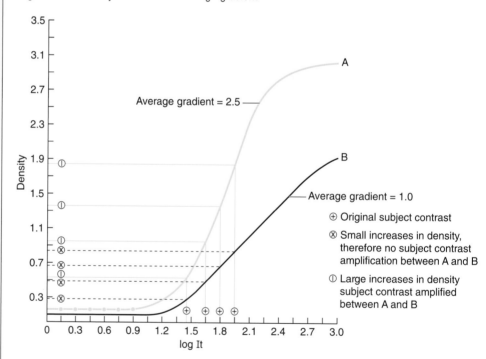 **Fig. E.8** Average gradient for two films, showing potential effect of subject contrast. **In Figure E.8** *Film A* • Average gradient 2.5 • Therefore an increase in subject contrast of 2.5 • Therefore large increases in density occur for relatively low increases in exposure

(continued on next page)

INFORMATION FROM THE CHARACTERISTIC CURVE *continued*

Final Contrast (contd)	*Film B* • Average gradient 1.0 • Therefore no increase in subject contrast • Therefore very small increases in density occur for the same increase in exposure as Film A • Therefore this film would not be suitable for medical radiography

Useful Exposure and Density Range	To determine the useful exposure range in Fig. E.9:
	• Net density 0.25 + base fog 0.16 = D 0.41
	• Net density 2.0 + base fog 0.16 = D 2.16
	• Vertical lines are drawn from the point where D 0.41 and 2.16 meet the characteristic curve
	• Area between the vertical lines determines:
	  ○ The latitude of the film (amount of over or under exposure a film will tolerate)
	  ○ Useful range of exposures (antilog It gives the mAs value) 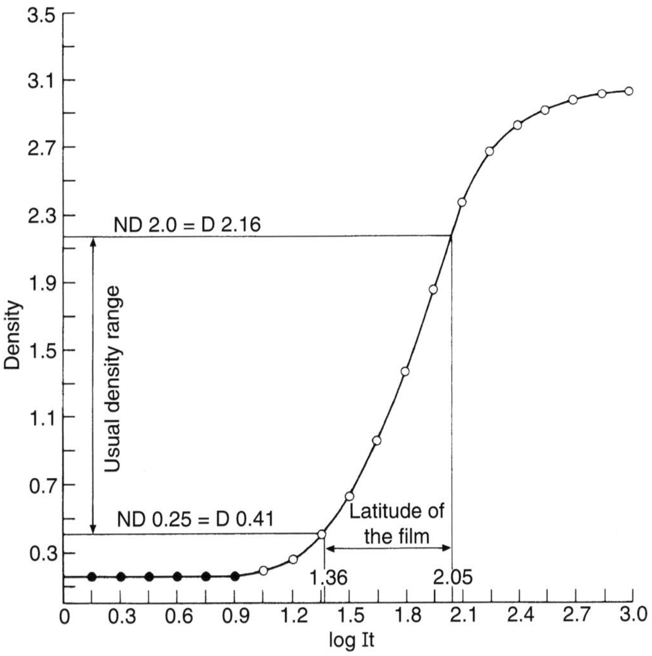
	
	Fig. E.9 Useful exposure and density range.

Fig. E.9 Useful exposure and density range.

(continued on next page)

INFORMATION FROM THE CHARACTERISTIC CURVE *continued*

Useful Exposure and Density Range (contd)

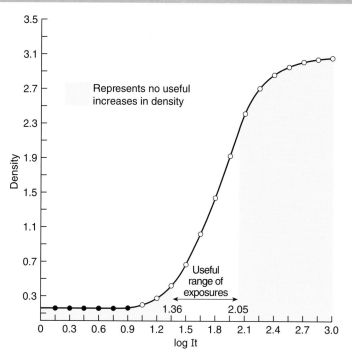

Fig. E.10 Small increase in exposure in the useful exposure range will increase density; below net density 0.25 and above net density 2.0 no noticeable change will occur for the same increase in exposure.

Application
- Log I/T 0.3 is equal to doubling (or halving) the exposure
- When setting automatic exposure devices they should be set to stop when the exposure reaches the mid-point of the straight line portion of the curve

Note
- The exposure latitude is linked to the average gradient of the film
  - The higher the average gradient, the lower the latitude of the film
  - The lower the average gradient, the higher the latitude

(continued on next page)

INFORMATION FROM THE CHARACTERISTIC CURVE *continued*

Speed	Speed = exposure required for a film to reach net density 1.0
	Usually, the nearer the density axis the faster the film because for a given exposure the film produces a higher density

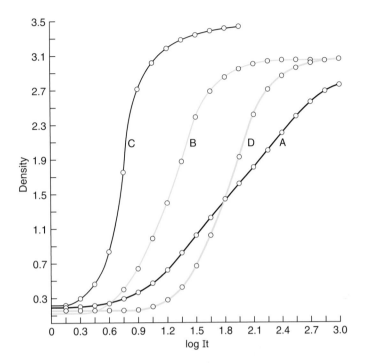

Fig. E.11 Comparisons of characteristic curves of four films.

In Figure E.11

Film A
- Not suitable for medical use
- Has average gradient of 1.0
- Faster than D below density 1.35
- Slower than D above density 1.35

Film B
- Identical to D except that B is faster
- B is slower than C

Film C
- Not suitable for medical use
- Has an unusable exposure latitude
- C is the fastest film

Film D
- Identical to B but is slower

(continued on next page)

INFORMATION FROM THE CHARACTERISTIC CURVE *continued*

Speed (*contd*)	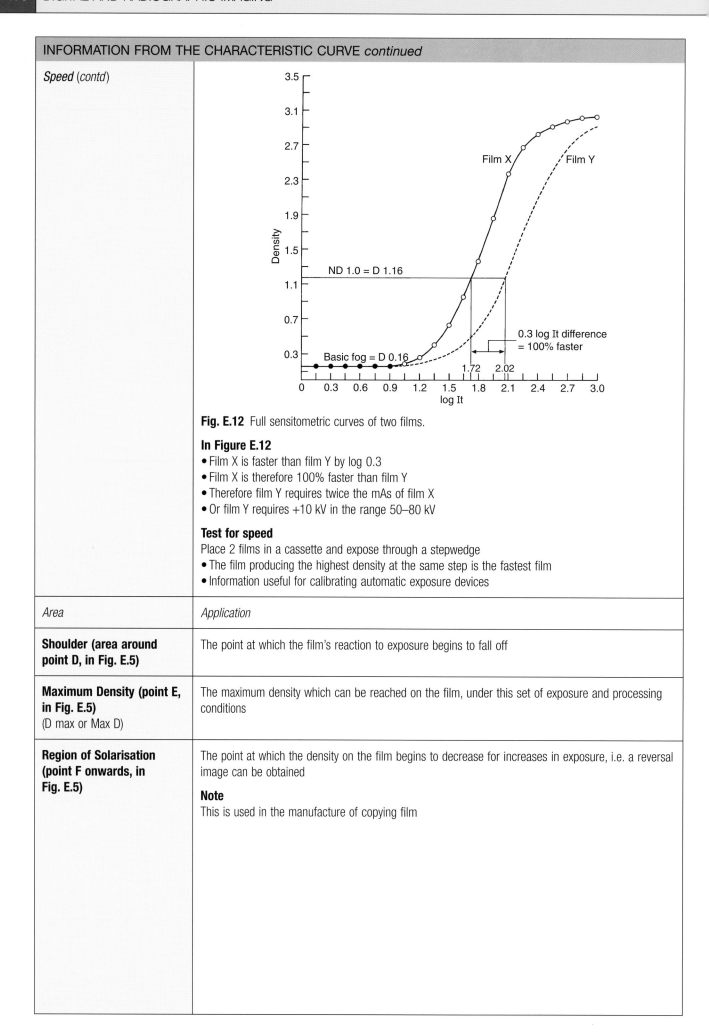

Fig. E.12 Full sensitometric curves of two films.

In Figure E.12
- Film X is faster than film Y by log 0.3
- Film X is therefore 100% faster than film Y
- Therefore film Y requires twice the mAs of film X
- Or film Y requires +10 kV in the range 50–80 kV

Test for speed
Place 2 films in a cassette and expose through a stepwedge
- The film producing the highest density at the same step is the fastest film
- Information useful for calibrating automatic exposure devices |

Area	Application
Shoulder (area around point D, in Fig. E.5)	The point at which the film's reaction to exposure begins to fall off
Maximum Density (point E, in Fig. E.5) (D max or Max D)	The maximum density which can be reached on the film, under this set of exposure and processing conditions
Region of Solarisation (point F onwards, in Fig. E.5)	The point at which the density on the film begins to decrease for increases in exposure, i.e. a reversal image can be obtained

Note
This is used in the manufacture of copying film |

QUALITY ASSURANCE	
	With the advent of the Ionising Regulations (1985) and the current EC directive, the onus is on department heads to prove that equipment is working correctly; quality assurance is a tool to provide that check

Quality Assurance	• A system to ensure that diagnostic images are of sufficiently high quality to provide adequate diagnostic information, with the least exposure of the patient to radiation and at the lowest possible cost
	• The objective is to monitor the performance of all the factors which could influence the quality of the image and to try to reduce any film wastage within that department
	• Wastage can be as high as 20%, with an average of 12%
	• If a quality assurance programme is designed for an imaging department it should ideally fulfil four main criteria:
	  ○ It should be quantitative, so that repeatability of results is assured
	  ○ It should be simple
	  ○ It should be inexpensive
	  ○ It should be quick
	• In a quality assurance programme it is important that the results achieved in January can be reproduced the following January

Reject Analysis
• Prior to starting quality assurance it is usual to do a study of reject analysis of film wastage (i.e. why were films repeated?)
• To establish the 'norm' for the department
• The longer the period for these analyses, the better the statistical values obtained
	Stage one
	• Inform *all* the staff that the survey is starting
	• The aims of the project should be stressed:
	  ○ To try to identify where, and why, the wastage is occurring
	  ○ To try to reduce the overall costs within the imaging department
	  ○ That the analysis is not a 'witch hunt', to identify poor radiographers, but is an assessment of the current conditions
	
	Stage two
	• A period of 8–10 weeks is set aside to conduct the survey, ideally starting on a Monday morning and finishing on a Friday night
	  ○ Prior to the start, all film in the department must be identified, counted and the details recorded
	  ○ The easiest way of achieving this is to empty all cassettes, the film hopper and any partially empty boxes. This film is then set aside until the end of the survey, when it can be subsequently used
	• To ensure accuracy of the records, a check must then be kept, on a daily basis, of all films removed from the film stores
	
	Stage three
	• Film analysis should be conducted on a daily basis
	• The rejected films should then be sorted out into categories

Suggested Categories	• Positioning • Movement • Too light • Too dark (unknown whether films are over- or under-exposed: may be machine/processor/screen problem) • Processing (marks, scratches, etc.) • Others (i.e. screen artefacts, light beam diaphragms, etc.) • Rejects by room
Analysis	At the end of each week: • All films remaining in the department are counted • The films used will be known, because of the record of movement of film from the film store • The total number of films used can be obtained • Calculate the percentage of films rejected • If the aim is to assess the wastage of film, calculate the total square meterage rejected. This figure gives a guide to the actual cost

(continued on next page)

QUALITY ASSURANCE *continued*

Analysis (contd)

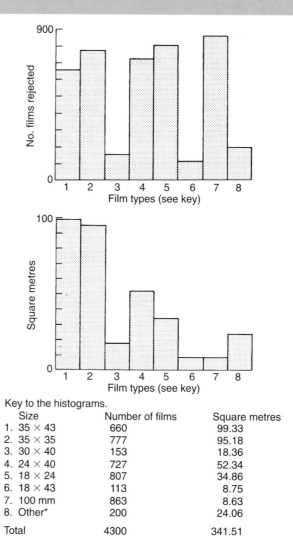

Key to the histograms.

Size	Number of films	Square metres
1. 35 × 43	660	99.33
2. 35 × 35	777	95.18
3. 30 × 40	153	18.36
4. 24 × 40	727	52.34
5. 18 × 24	807	34.86
6. 18 × 43	113	8.75
7. 100 mm	863	8.63
8. Other*	200	24.06
Total	4300	341.51

* CT, duplicating film, copy films, occlusals, etc.

Fig. F.1 Presentation of statistics obtained from a reject analysis survey.

Note

Ten 18 × 24 films do not represent the same cost as ten 35 × 43 films

Square meterage per box of 100 films

Film size (×100)	Square metres
13 × 18 cm	2.34
15 × 40 cm	6.00
18 × 24 cm	4.32
20 × 40 cm	8.00
24 × 30 cm	7.20
30 × 40 cm	12.00
35 × 35 cm	12.25
35 × 43 cm	15.05
6½ × 8½ in	3.56
8 × 10 in	5.16
10 × 12 in	7.75
12 × 15 in	11.62
7 × 17 in	7.74
15 × 6 in	5.79

(continued on next page)

QUALITY ASSURANCE *continued*

Information Gained	• Rooms which may be consistently faulty • Poor technique indicating a training need • Cassettes and screens may be identified which are outside speed tolerances • Cost of running the department • Need for extra staff
Information Unrecorded	**Diagnostic criteria** • When a radiographer accepts a film, even though it would normally be unacceptable, because it would be very difficult or impossible to repeat it **Compensation** • When the radiographer compensates for an already known fault

QUALITY ASSURANCE PROGRAMMES

	Involve regular monitoring of:
Image Producers	• X-ray set • Associated equipment • Could include the image intensifier, ect.
Image Receptors	• X-ray intensifying screens • X-ray film • Television monitors
Image Processors	• Processing machine found in the imaging department
Viewing System	• Conventional viewing boxes

APPARATUS REQUIRED

A Densitometer	See sensitometry p. 163
A Contact Test Grid	For testing cassettes for screen film contact **Fig. F.2** A contact test grid.
An Ultraviolet Light The output to be 250 Nm or below	For testing cassettes and screens

(continued on next page)

APPARATUS REQUIRED *continued*	
A Calibrated Step Wedge or **A Sensitometer** or **Manufacturer's Pre-Exposed Step Wedge Film** or **Computerised Processor Control**	See sensitometry p. 162
Alcohol Thermometer, plus a Maximum–Minimum Thermometer	• Used for direct measurements of solution temperatures • A mercury thermometer is *not* recommended as breakages can cause photographic faults
Hydrometer	Measures specific gravity • Too low, then the solutions are too dilute, i.e. somehow too much water has been added • Too high, not enough water has been added
A Ph Meter	To measure pH • Check correct replenishment rates of developer and fixer • Measured daily • Developers range between 9.0 and 10.6 • Fixers range between 4.0 and 5.0
Silver Estimating Papers	Give a guide of the quantity of silver in the fixer in grams per litre (g/1) • When these papers are placed in fixer they change colour • Colour change is matched against a colour chart • Level should be about 6–7 g of silver per litre of fixer • Too high a silver level can be caused by under-replenishment and will result in incomplete fixing of the film • A typical processor will contain about 120–140 g of silver, which is all recoverable
Replenishment Rate Checks	**Gross over-replenishment of developer** • Gradual increase of pH • The basic fog will begin to rise **Fig. F.3** Developer grossly over-replenished. **Gross under-replenishment of developer** • Causes the pH to drop • Maximum densities are not reached on the film • Apparent decrease in the film's speed

(continued on next page)

APPARATUS REQUIRED *continued*

Replenishment Rate Checks
(*contd*)

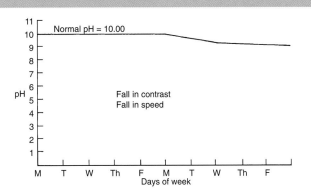

Fig. F.4 Developer grossly under-replenished.

Gross under-replenishment of fixer
- The pH now increases
- Transport problems due to the film swelling excessively in the wash water because of inadequate hardening
- Scratches due to a very soft non-hardened emulsion
- Non-drying because of excess water in the emulsion
- A fall in average gradient due to a milky white overall fog shown on the film due to non-fixation

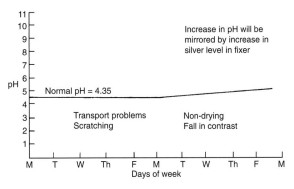

Fig. F.5 Fixer grossly under-replenished.

EQUIPMENT TESTS

Safelights

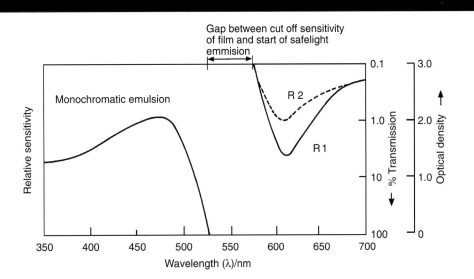

Fig. F.6 Safelight transmission features versus film spectral sensitivity, showing a 'safe' combination with two different safelight filters: R1 and R2.

(*continued on next page*)

EQUIPMENT TESTS *continued*

Function To provide a high level of 'darkroom' illumination without any detrimental effect on the sensitive material (film)	**Principles of operation** The selective optical filtering of a white light source so the film material is subject only to wavelengths to which it is not sensitive The performance of a particular filter can be assessed by plotting the percentage of light transmitted through the filter at selected wavelengths • For monochromatic emulsions an orange safelight • For orthochromatic a dark red safelight • For panchromatic total darkness
Factors Affecting Safelight Performance	**Distance and bulb wattage** The higher the wattage, the further away it needs to be 'safe' (inverse square law applies) • For a direct safelight with a 25 W bulb, the closet distance is 1.2 m • For an indirect safelight, i.e. one that depends entirely on reflection from the walls and ceiling up to a 60 W bulb **Number and position** • One indirect light for every 6 m^2 of ceiling area at a height of 2 m above floor level for a general level of illumination • Too many and/or badly positioned safelights can have an effect on the base + fog level of the film **White light leakage** A cracked or damaged filter or housing may be sufficient to raise the base + fog level **Safe handling time** This is the length of time the film may be handled in normal safelight conditions without an increase in the base + fog level • Approximately 45 seconds
Testing The International Organisation for Standardisation (ISO) Safelight test	**ISO 8374 – Photography – Determination of ISO safelight conditions (December 1986)** Contains a full description of the pre-exposure, post-exposure tests and the test used during the processing cycle, along with a glossary of definitions
Test Equipment	• A pre-exposed step tablet, or • The film is loaded into a cassette and an exposure of 5 mAs and 40 kV, is given • The film is covered with strips of card, ensuring that the top 2.5 cm strip of the film remains covered and therefore unexposed • The following 2.5 cm strips are uncovered in turn and each strip is given an exposure (using a light of the same spectral quality as that of the intensifying screens) using a series of exposure times (e.g. 1 s, 2 s, 4 s, 8 s, 16 s, 32 s, etc.) and using the card to uncover a different strip of film for each exposure • When processed it would look as if it had been made by using a step wedge
Data Recording A record should be kept of all pertinent data	• Safelight filter designation • Size • Age • Lamp type • Wattage and voltage • Distance from filter to film • Sensitised film type • Safelight exposure times • Processing data
Testing the Safelights	• The 'step wedge' film is placed on the bench in total darkness • The film is covered with two pieces of card ensuring the left (or right 2.5 cm strip of the film remains covered and therefore unexposed (this strip will include an image of all the 'steps' of the step wedge and will be used for comparison purposes) • The following 2.5 cm strips are uncovered in turn

(continued on next page)

EQUIPMENT TESTS *continued*

Testing the Safelights (contd)	• Each strip is given an exposure to the safelights, each exposure time being increased by a factor of 2 (e.g. 4 s, 8 s, 16 s, 32 s, etc.) and using the card to uncover a different strip of film for each exposure • The film is processed
Evaluation	• The densities of all the strips are measured • The density of the strips which have been exposed to safelights are compared with the strip which was not exposed to safelights • The strip which received the most safelight exposure without increasing the density of any step is determined • The exposure time of this final strip is then divided by 2, giving the 'ISO safelight condition'

FILM

Stock Control	All film has a 'shelf life' • When films are received into the department they should be date stamped, or identified in some way so that the date of entry into the department is known • They should be used in strict rotation
Storage Conditions	• Store film vertically, not horizontally, to prevent pressure marks • An even temperature in the order of 10°C • 50% relative humidity • Store away from photographic chemicals • Certain fumes are known to fog films, e.g. carbon monoxide, formalin and formaldehyde, certain types of paint and mercury vapour • Avoid some building materials like breeze block, as some constituents may be minutely radioactive

INTENSIFYING SCREENS AND CASSETTES

Numbering	• Number cassettes, both inside and out • This enables the identification of a faulty screen or cassette
Routine Cleaning	• Only clean screens with the cleaning solution recommended by the manufacturer of the screens • Dust and dirt should be removed with a soft brush, such as a camera lens cleaning brush • For ingrained dirt, use a lint-free cloth and screen cleaner, rubbing in a circular motion without undue pressure • Once the screens have been cleaned, leave the cassettes partially open so the screens can dry naturally **Note** Most screen cleaners contain an antistatic element. Static will attract dirt and dust
Inspection	• Inspect by reflected white light • Any bad surface marks and scratches will usually show up • Any screens with marks in the central area should go for further tests • When scanned with the UV light, in an unlit room, the surface phosphors are excited and artefacts and abrasions can be seen
Screen Contact Test British Standard: The test for screen contact is covered by British Standard, BS7725-2.2 1994, and IEC 61223-2-2 1993. These standards cover cassettes, film changers and film screen contact	**Test method** • One cassette, ideally of a small format, should be chosen as a control cassette • This cassette, loaded with film, should be placed in the centre of every group of cassettes of the same speed class, which is exposed during the tests. The control cassette will act as confirmation of reproducibility • The same density should be recorded on this control cassette after every exposure • A record should be kept of the position of every cassette during the tests. If density variations are found from 'north' to 'south', but are similar in all test exposures, the variations can be assumed to be caused by the anode heel effect

(continued on next page)

INTENSIFYING SCREENS AND CASSETTES *continued*

Screen Contact Test (contd)	• The test tool is placed on top of the cassette and the beam is centred to the centre of the cassette and test tool • The film is exposed using 50 kV, 1.00 or 1.5 mm focal spot, a distance of 1.5 m • Sufficient mAs to produce a density of between 2.00 and 3.00 as this is used for the speed measurements • The film is processed and viewed at a distance of 4 m as it is impossible to see the defects at close range • A cassette with good screen contact produces films with an overall even density • Poor contact shows up as patches of high density areas • Cassettes that show poor screen contact in the central area should be rejected. Loss of contact in other areas should be evaluated by the individuals concerned 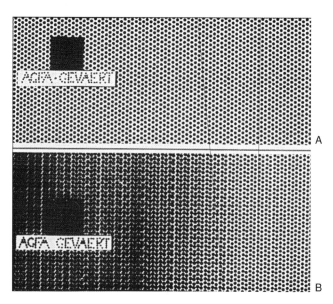 **Fig. F.7** (A) Radiograph produced by a cassette with good screen contact. (B) Radiograph produced by a cassette with poor screen contact.
Speed Tests	• A density of greater than 2.0 is produced in the central area of the film • The density of the central cut out is measured and all the values recorded for each of the cassettes tested. • The average is then taken of the highest density values recorded within every speed class • Cassettes which have recorded significantly less than this average density should be rejected on grounds of unacceptable speed loss **Note** If, for example, the densities recorded on a class 200 approach class 100 densities, then the cassette can be rejected in terms of speed achievement and re-allocated as a class 100
Light Leakage Light leakage will be well demonstrated by areas of fogging along the edge of films	• Using an 100 Watt tungsten lamp expose each edge of the cassette, the front and the back, for 15 minutes using a distance of 1.22 m • A total of 6 exposures taking one and a half hours • An edge darkening of more than 3.2 mm on the exposed film is significant

THE VIEWING SYSTEM

Viewing Box Evaluation • To achieve correct and constant light output throughout the department • To achieve the correct balance between viewer light output and the ambient light in the viewing room	**Test equipment** A specifically designed unit which consists of: • A hand held optical recorder • Laser beam to allow for correct positioning • A mechanical distance indicator • Digital display giving a reading in candela per square meter • The ability to store the data recorded • The unit is used to assess the overall light intensity from a specific viewing box so that comparisons can be made between viewing boxes to ensure standardisation of viewing facilities
Cleaning	• Both outside and inside • Using anti-static polish
Colour Temperature	• Most X-ray films used in the department have a blue base • Therefore use fluorescent tubes with a wavelength of about 6500 K • 'Northern Light' or 'Tropical Daylight', both produce bright, 'blue/ white' light **Note** If one tube fails it is better to change all the tubes in the viewing box

CHEMICALS IN THE ENVIRONMENT

	The advent of computerisation and imaging plates enabling the electronic transfer of information saves on silver-containing film, and reduction in film processing and chemical usage. But, for a few departments, the conventional use of films and processing still continue and this appendix will concentrate on the impact of chemicals in the environment

THE CONTROL OF CHEMICAL POLLUTION

Air Pollution	See COSHH Regulations, p. 108 to 109
Soil Pollution by Solid Bodies	Not applicable
Water Pollution	**pH values** • The pH of the developer (is approximately 10) • The pH of the fixer (approximately 4.5) • If they are discharged, with the wash water, the pH of the effluent will be in the alkaline rather than the unwanted acid range

CHEMICAL POLLUTION FACTORS

Poisonous materials	• Substances which kill organisms living in the water
Biologically Oxidisable Material	• When these substances are decomposed by micro-organisms living in the water oxygen is consumed • Therefore aquatic and vegetable life cannot exist
Nutrients	• Upset the ecological balance by promoting the uncontrolled growth of plants and algae
BOD5 (Biological Oxygen Demand 5)	• The number of milligrams of oxygen, consumed over 5 days, per litre of waste water • A sample of water is collected and the oxygen content is measured – • The water is incubated at 20°C for 5 days and the oxygen content is measured – • By calculating the difference between the two amounts the BOD can be calculated
Effluent	• If a newly installed processor is connected to a foul sewer a trade effluent consent must be obtained from the local Water Authority • Some rural hospitals have their own treatment works and therefore the National Rivers Authority should be contacted as the final effluent may enter surface water channels • The trade effluent consent would specify the amount of discharge permitted including the amount of silver in parts per million

THE MAIN PHOTOGRAPHIC POLLUTANTS

Metals Many metallic ions have a serious effect on micro-organisms and fish	None of these should be discharged into sewerage systems
Silver	• A silver ion it is very toxic for most micro-organisms and fish • Silver in the waste water is found as a thiosulphate compound from the wash water • Any silver ions present will form almost insoluble salts when combined with chloride, bromide and sulphide ions which are normally present in waste water • See the Water Act, p. 109 • The effluent from any silver recovery unit is monitored on a regular basis to check that no silver is being discharged from the unit • The manager of an imaging department is responsible for ensuring that if a bulk collection service is used, the company is reputable and are licensed to dispose of the solutions

POSSIBLE CHEMICAL CONTAMINANTS

Phenols 1 mg of hydroquinone per litre of water can prove toxic for some fish	• Hydroquinone is a phenol derivative • If hydroquinone is discharged into a surface water channel the concentration should be kept low
Ammoniacal Nitrogen	• In fixer, ammonium ions are used • Free ammonia can only occur in an alkaline medium • As used fixer is mixed with the developer and waste water the resultant effluent is alkaline
Organic Solvents	• These are diluted to make processing solution • They are then diluted in waste water • Therefore only small traces remain
Nutrients	• The majority of phosphates and nitrates have been eliminated from processing solutions

Oxidising Agents
• Developer and sodium sulphite (used to prevent oxidation of the developer) will increase BOD5
• Fixer contains thiosulphate, sulphite which is easily oxidisable
• Waste water is mixed with waste developer and fixer
	• Replenishment of both developer and fixer cause contamination of the waste water
	• Developer replenishment should be optimised
	• Fixer recycled
	• Fixer replenishment is minimised
	• Wash water can be recycled, saving 75% of water used
	  ○ As the water has been heated there is an energy saving
	  ○ And the amount of silver discharged is negligible
	• Waste water discharge should be evenly distributed during the day, and may need a collection tank so that it can drain slowly

Books

Ball J, Price T 1995 Chesney's radiographic imaging. Blackwell Science, London

Boden L 1995 Mastering CD-Rom technology. John Wiley, Oxford

Bushong S C 2004 Radiologic science for technologists, 8th edn. Elsevier Mosby, St Louis

Carlton R R, Adler A M 1996 Principles of radiographic imaging. Delmar, London

Carter P H 1994 Chesney's equipment for student radiographers. Blackwell Science, London

College of Radiographers and the British Association of MR Radiographers 2002 Safety issues in magnetic resonance imaging: guidance for radiographers. London

Davis A, Fennessy P 1994 Electronic imaging for photographers. Focal Press, Oxford

Dol K, Macmahon H, Giger M L, Hoffman K R 1998 Computer aided diagnosis in medical imaging. Elsevier, Amsterdam

Fauber T L 2000 Radiographic imaging and exposure. Mosby, St Louis

Gonzales R C, Woods R E 1992 Digital image processing. Addison Wesley, Wokingham

Graham D T 1996 Principles of radiological physics. Churchill Livingstone, Edinburgh

Graham R 1998 Digital imaging. Whittles, Scotland

Greenfield G B, Hubbard L B 1984 Computers in radiology. Churchill Livingstone, Edinburgh

Hajinal J V, Hill D L G, Hawkes D J 2001 Medical image registration. CRC Press, London

Hashemi R H, Bradley W G, Lisanti C J 2003 MRI: The Basics, 2nd edn. Wolters Kluwer, London

Hornak J 2002 The basics of MRI. RIT, Rochester

Huang H 1996 PACS: Picture archiving and communication systems in biomedical imaging. VCH, New York

Oakley J 2003 Digital imaging.Cambridge University Press, Cambridge

Pizzutiello R J 1993 Introduction to medical radiographic imaging. Eastman Kodak, New York

Russ J C 1998 The image processing handbook. CRC Press, London

Sanders R C 1991 Clinical sonography – a practical guide, 2nd edn. Little Brown, Boston

Stockley S M 1986 A manual of radiographic equipment. Churchill Livingstone, Edinburgh

Sutton D 1988 Radiology and imaging for medical students. Churchill Livingstone, Edinburgh

Sutton D 2002 Textbook of radiology and imaging, Vol 2, 7th edn. Churchill Livingstone, Edinburgh

Watteville A, Naughton S 1998 Advanced information technology. Heinemann GNVQ, Oxford

Webb W R, Brant W E, Helms C A 1998 Fundamentals of body CT, 2nd edn. Saunders, Philadelphia

Westbrook C, Kaut Roth, C 1993 MRI in practice. Blackwell Scientific, London

Wilson B 1996 Information technology – the basics. City and Guilds/Macmillan, London

Websites

http://DICOM.nema.org
www.adaclabs.com
www.agfa.com/healthcare
www.agocg.ac.uk
www.amershamhealth.com
www.analog.com
www.answers.com
www.anzai-medical.com
www.bkmed.com
www.carestreamhealth.com
www.cs.swan.ac.uk
www.digirad.com
www.emedialive.com
www.es.oersted.dtu.dk
www.fonar.com
www.fujifilm.com
www.gal.ac.com
www.gehealthcare.com
www.hitachi-medical-systems.com
www.howstuffworks.com
www.imagingmanagement.org
www.imaginis.com
www.isotrak.de
www.latticesemi.com
www.maxim-ic.com
www.medial.siemens.com

(continued on next page)

www.medical.philips.com/uk
www.osta.org/technology
www.picker.com
www.sectra.com
www.shimadzu.com
www.siemens.com/nmg
www.studentbmj.com
www.techworld.com
www.toshiba-europe.com/medical